Attracting Your Perfect Body
through the Chakras

by Cyndi Dale

CROSSING PRESS
Berkeley

All rights reserved. Published in the United States by Crossing Press, an imprint of Corwn Publishing Group, a division of Random House, Inc., New York.
www.crownpublishing.com
www.tenspeed.com

Crossing Press and the Crossing Press colophon are registered trademarks of Random House, Inc.

Library of Congress Cataloging-in-Publication Data
Dale, Cyndi.
  Attracting your perfect body through the chakras / by Cyndi Dale.
   p. cm.
  1. Physical fitness--Psychological aspects. 2. Chakras.   I. Title.
   GV481.2.D35 2006
   613.7'046--dc22

                    2005034054

ISBN: 978-1-58091-174-0

Printed in the U.S.A.

Cover design by Katy Brown
Text design by Lisa Buckley
Front cover photo by Brand X Pictures/Media Bakery

10 9 8 7 6 5 4 3 2

First Edition

Contents

Introduction:
The Key to Your Perfect Body

Your perfect body already lies inside of you! You are only a few steps away from looking into the mirror and seeing it.

Are you overweight? Your trim self exists within the armor forged of too many candy bars or mashed potatoes. Do you think you are a bit too skinny? Your toned, muscle-built self is like a deflated balloon; it just needs a little helium. Underneath everything that you do not like about your body is a perfectly fit, likable body. You just have to find the key that will unlock it.

What is the secret? *Personalizing the process.* No one else has your perfect body. For that matter, no one else can follow your path to perfection, either.

Of the innumerable snowflakes that fall each year, no two are the same. Glance at magazines, the products at the pharmacy, or advertisements, however, and you will find nothing but generic approaches for creating the perfect body. "Drink nothing but our special concoction and in five weeks you'll have lost 100 pounds," asserts one diet company. "Pray in this position (after sending us a contribution), and God will remove your defects," vows yet another expert. "Exercise with our complicated and expensive contraption and you'll have tight abdominal muscles," boasts another. Whether the formula requires counting carbohydrates or prayers, restricting fats or fun, or figuring out whether you are shaped like a pear, an apple, or a Christmas tree, it is supposed to work for everyone.

It does not work that way.

The fundamentals of your *physical* body are encoded in your genes. However, the formula for your *perfect* body is scripted on a different set of genes, one that is made of energy. Your chakras are encoded for your perfect body.

Chakras are energy organs. Even though you cannot see, touch, or hear your chakras, except with special techniques and tools, they are as real as your heart or your brain, and they can help you transform your *current body* into your *perfect body.*

There are countless chakras, but the primary eleven rule your physical body and well-being. Chakras change physical matter into spiritual energy and vice versa. They can convert a solid lump of fat into smooth muscle. They can put a glow on your skin and happiness in your heart. By deciphering the information in your chakras, you can determine which fashions and colors best match your personality and enhance your appearance, which exercise will sculpt the perfect you, and which foods are potentially suited for transforming yourself into a model of fitness and health.

By following the formulas encoded in your chakras, you can release your perfect body, the body that reveals your real self. Your perfect body will not be identical to those of swimsuit models or body builders. *Instead, your perfect body will be the body that is perfect for you.* It will be full of life energy. It will attract relationships that make you joyous, and it will put a spring in your step. Your perfect body will allow you to present your best face to the world and attract your perfect job opportunities. And when you reveal all your assets to the world, the world will respond in kind with love and support.

To uncover the formula for your perfect body and put it into practice, you have only to determine your chakric strengths and weaknesses. Everyone has the same number and location of chakras, but some of your chakras are stronger than others. By identifying and magnetizing your strongest chakras, you flood your body with the energy you need to become healthy and fit. By understanding the information provided by these chakras, you can build a plan for healthy living.

1

You Have Tried It All: Why Has Nothing Worked?

> Merlinnus turned and said quietly,
> "It is not what I believe, Gawen. It is what I know.
> There are many truths. A priest's truth may not
> be a king's truth. A king's truth may not be
> a kingdom's truth."
>
> Jane Yolen, *Sword of the Rightful King*

The Quest for the Perfect Body

Don't look now, but your fairy godmother has flown into the room where you are sitting, reading this book.

"Dear," she says, waving her magic wand. "I am giving you one wish. You have to use it to better your body. What will it be? Hurry up now," she adds, with a glance at her watch. "I don't have all day."

What would you choose? Would it be tighter abdominal muscles, bulging biceps, fresher skin, or maybe toned thighs? Many of us would opt for a whole new look, an entirely renovated self.

Maybe you are one of the few people who is entirely pleased with her body, but I doubt it. More than 60 percent of all Americans (and 50 percent of children) are now overweight, and this trend is not confined to the United States. The World Health Organization has coined a new word—*globesity*—that suggests the immensity of the problem.

Consider the billions of dollars spent each year on exercise and weight loss programs, skin care, personal grooming, plastic surgery, and other cosmetic care, and the depth of despair most of us feel about our appearance becomes clear. We assume that if we looked a little leaner, sexier, more muscular, or more glamorous—more *perfect*—we would be happier and more successful. Well, we might be! However, we will only be satisfied—even thrilled—with our appearance if we summon forth the body that is personally perfect for us. This means contemplating the real reason that we want a perfect body. We yearn for a perfect body because we want a perfect life.

The Desire for the Perfect Life

The desire for the perfect body is synonymous with the wish for a perfect life. Deep inside, most of us have a fairy tale about what the "perfect" life looks and feels like. It might involve anything from living in a castle (or large house), to getting to eat our favorite foods all the time, to having a magic closet that always contains the perfect outfit for us to wear. But these fairy tales are confusing (not to mention staggering financially).

None of us lives up to the plastic images established by the media, culture, or our own perfectionist standards. Moreover, as you might suspect, those who look so perfect in pictures do not actually look like their photographs. It is said that the camera doesn't lie, but that doesn't mean advertisers don't. It is only possible to create a flawless body through airbrushing and illusion.

To be "perfect" you don't have to look flawless or be free from shortcomings. "Perfection," instead, can indicate a state of completion. When we are complete, we do not lack anything essential. A big house might not really be essential to living a happy life. Nor is it necessary to have a nose or biceps of a certain size. Having a perfect life or perfect body is not about living up to a fixed set of standards. Instead, it involves living a life that is perfect for you, within a body that is perfectly designed by your most "perfect self," your spirit.

THE SPIRITUAL PROMISE OF THE GOOD LIFE

Spiritual truths across many cultures emphasize the importance of living a happy and joyous life, achieved partly through bodily pleasures. Ecclesiastes 3:12–13 states, "I know that there is nothing better for them than to be happy and enjoy themselves as long as they live; also that it is God's gift to man that everyone should eat and drink and take pleasure in all his toil." The ancient Maya also believed in enjoying the bounty of life. Mayan expert Hunbatz Men writes, "If the departed has earned a reward, it is here on Earth that it will be enjoyed."[1] And, according to the way of Shambhala, a universal warrior code, we must never forget the goodness of this world, and the wonder and necessity of living fully.

You can—and should—live fully right now, even if you are overweight or out of shape, or maybe just dissatisfied with your nose, your hair, or your appearance in general. You are a diamond. You are already perfect, because you are already your essence, that perfect reflection of the Divine that is here to experience imperfection in all its grace and beauty.

ATTRACTING YOUR PERFECT BODY BY OWNING YOUR PERFECTION

Whatever the state of your body, you are already in possession of perfection: *It is perfect that you are alive at this time in history.*

You are here on purpose. The Divine and all other beings on this planet and in the cosmos are in clear agreement. You are supposed to be alive right now. The universe depends upon your fulfilling a vital, singular mission, and you need your physical body to meet your goals and fulfill your purpose.

You are destined to play a role in the drama of the universe. This role is to express at least one spiritual truth throughout everything that you do, think, and say. By sharing your truth, you change the world. You invite the world to unfold its greatness, even as you do the same.

Spiritual truths differ from everyday truths in that they focus on higher ideals, like truth, faith, and joy. Some of us express similar spiritual truths, but because we have different personalities, we will reflect these truths differently. This means that *what* we communicate and *how* we communicate are both universal and distinctive.

To express your truth to the world, you are blessed with specific attributes and abilities that are unique to you. Your essential truth and supportive gifts are encoded in your spirit or essence, the spark of the Divine that reflects the "you" that is perfectly "you." Your spirit has programmed its truths and your gifts into every aspect of your being, including your body. This means that your body is actually designed to help you fulfill your spiritual purpose. *Therefore, your perfect body is the body that enables you most fully to live your unique spiritual purpose and access your special spiritual gifts.*

Fulfilling your life mission might not require a tiny figure if you are a woman, or a set of toned abdominal muscles if you are a man. Let's assume that you are to be an expression of divine truth through singing. Your body will be equipped with the correct genetics to make you an effective opera singer. You will have a solid diaphragm, broad shoulders, and a tall frame. Or perhaps your mission is to heal through the chiropractic arts. You will require strong arms, an even stronger back, and a logical mind.

To best be able to carry out your mission and access your gifts, you will need to follow the specific types of regimens that support your real self. You will need to adopt the behaviors, attitudes, and style that reflect your spiritual essence. This way, your body can be the vehicle for your spirit that it was meant to be.

Life is full of challenges. Perhaps you were not raised to feel good about yourself. Then you probably have not fully claimed your purpose or tended to your body in order to perfect it. This book will help you do both. Maybe emotional or psychological wounds have kept you from claiming your right to your spiritually perfect body. You might need therapeutic or medical support to work through these issues, in which case this book would serve as a supplement to those practices. Whatever your current state, know this: At any time you can begin or accelerate the process of summoning your perfect body from deep inside your tissues and flesh. You can beckon your perfect body from its hiding place under your bones. Moreover, you can learn how to attract powerful energies from the heavens to forge and maintain your perfect body.

EXERCISE: BEING YOURSELF

Think back to a time when you felt completely comfortable with your body. You loved every inch of your physical self and felt good being in your own skin. Now remember the circumstances around this self-acceptance. What factors allowed this level of acceptance? Were there other individuals involved, and if so, in what way? What inner messages were supporting your confidence? What other reasons were you holding yourself in such high esteem? How had you recently treated your body? How were you eating, dressing, moving, or interacting with others?

Now make a list of the factors contributing to your self-acceptance, grouping them under the following headings: physical, emotional, mental, and spiritual. See if you can reduce each of the four lists to one or two sentences. For example, under the heading "spiritual" you might write, "Believed myself loved by the Divine." Under physical, you might pinpoint, "Wore clothes that expressed my creativity." Reflect upon your findings, and ask yourself how you might incorporate these beliefs or behaviors into your everyday life.

2
Your Body as Energy

"Consciousness was the first thing in that terrifying explosion of matter and energy that God recognized as being like himself."

"That's what God is? Awareness?"

"I think so . . . Pure information."

Greg Iles, *The Footprints of God*

Your Body as Information

To achieve your perfect body, you must understand that your body is made of energy. In fact, your body is a swirling composite of various types, colors, tones, and shapes of energy.

All energy contains information. The information in a rose tells the rose to be a rose. The information called "memory" is largely responsible for creating the "you" that you are today. Of course, nothing in the world is static. Even a motionless rose is constantly moving, as is every cell in your body. Different types of information vibrate at different rates. When you add information and vibration, you arrive at the actual definition of the word "energy." Energy is vibrating information. The only way to attract your perfect body is to do so energetically, because your body is made of energy.

The image of yourself that you see in the mirror is composed of one type of energy particle. These particles are quarks, the basis of sensory reality. Sensory reality consists of the things you can see, touch, hear, and measure. It is the reality that you studied in school. When you have coffee with a friend, your conversation is a sensory-based communication. Quarks are the tiny subatomic particles that carry information at a vibrational frequency that is understandable to your five senses. Their vibratory rate is relatively low, slower than the speed of light.

In addition to quarks, the world is populated by another set of subatomic particles, called tachyons. Tachyons, which move faster than the speed of light, underlie psychic reality, or spiritual reality. Psychic reality is not as confining as sensory reality. When you are dealing with psychic energy, you can receive information from the past, the present, or the potential future. Because psychic energy moves faster than the speed of light, it does not have to obey normal laws. Relating with a friend over coffee, using psychic energy, you can hear her next words before she utters them, or finish your coffee before you have even started it. A talented psychic person could change an ordinary cup of coffee into an exotic drink with just a wish.

Because tachyons vibrate at extremely high frequencies, they are difficult to tune into through traditional means. And because of the challenge of "proving" psychic phenomena, they are often called "paranormal" or "supernatural." Psychic reality, however, is really an extension of the world of the spirit and spirituality. In fact, a lot of your innate psychic information comes from your internal spirit, and thus lies at the core of your perfect body.

Your current body is primarily made of the sensory information that comes from your genes, family of origin, culture, and experiences. Your perfect body is a reflection of the psychic information that emanates from your spirit. The reason that I call this book *Attracting Your Perfect Body* instead of *Creating Your Perfect Body* is that the easiest way to realize your ideal physical body is to base your conditioning program on your psychically known spiritual needs, codes, truths, and programs. By taking practical steps with your spirit in mind, you accelerate your fitness regime and speed the integration of your spirit with your body. In addition, you attract universal energies that can accelerate your perfect development.

Of course, you have to take the everyday, practical steps necessary to lose weight, optimize your fitness, and appear your best. There are no shortcuts, only ways to move faster! Neither quarks nor tachyons are supernatural. There are natural laws governing how each operates. However, there is something miraculous about combining these two forces in your life. By allowing your quarks and tachyons to work together, you can create the body that you are supposed to have.

Quark versus Tachyon Fitness Program

If you have ever been on a traditional diet, then you have followed a "quark" plan. To lose weight the quark way, you have to count calories (a measurement of energy), weigh your food portions, and exercise more so that you burn more calories than you consume. We have all tried this. It is a pretty slow process—and that's because quarks are slow.

A tachyon diet looks different from a quark diet. While your quark-self is chewing on carrots and lifting weights, your tachyon-self might be munching positive thoughts and weighing possible futures. Obtaining your perfect body will take both quark and tachyon efforts; it will necessitate behavioral *and* spiritual changes.

Your current body is anchored to present-day reality by sensory means, such as the amount you exercise or the foods you eat. If you want to alter your physical body, you will have to change your behavior. You will need to adopt actions that will rid you of negative sensory energies (like overweight or sloth) and help you maintain new standards (like healthy eating and fun exercise).

But it is also import to work the tachyon side of your perfect body program. Problems with your body are often secured by thoughts, beliefs, and feelings that are psychic in nature. The most common culprits are negative and self-defeating beliefs and repressed feelings.

A program for attracting the perfect body will summon forth your psychic or spiritual self, as well as attract spiritual energies that will help you sustain the program for the duration of your physical life. Your perfect body might partially inhabit the concrete world already. You are born with a certain bone structure, for example, and it is important to trust that this is the one most capable of helping you fulfill your spiritual promise. Other parts of your perfect body, however, might still be in disguise, locked into the realm of possibilities by certain psychic energies or physical actions.

Attracting your perfect body, then, is going to require two types of action:

1. You have to change your behavior. This is the quark part of your perfect body fitness program.
2. You have to work psychically or spiritually. This is the tachyon side of following your perfect body plan.

How do you create this magical fitness program? It's simple. You work with your chakras.

Your Energy System: Portals into the Perfect Body

Your chakras are the key to your perfect body program. Through these energy centers, you can purge a negative thought and then, poof—you eliminate the unconstructive energy holding onto a pound of fat. It works in the reverse, too. You can move your muscles and increase your self-esteem. By better understanding your chakras, you can construct your own quark *and* tachyon fitness program.

Chakras are the vital set of energy centers in your greater energy system. They are also called energy organs, because they work similarly to your physical organs. Your chakras work with energies both inside and outside of your body, assisting your spirit to achieve its destiny. Other energy centers support your destiny as well, but function slightly differently. We will concern ourselves later with one of these types of centers, the auric field, which plays an important role in establishing and maintaining the ideal body.

Your chakras are nourished by light and also emit light. In the white light spectrum, there are several colors. Each unique color is a different frequency and contains different types of information. In addition, each chakra has a unique frequency and governs certain types of life concerns. Like energy attracts like, which means that each chakra will attract the colored light or informed vibration that matches it. The term "informed energy" relates to our working definition of energy as "information that vibrates." Chakras are in the business of attracting, interpreting, and dissemination vibrating data. This means that if there are energies that should leave your body, such as negative thoughts or physical toxins, a chakra will spin this energy out of your body and back into the universe.

Through your chakras and energy organs, you can support the unfolding of your spirit's ideal body while attracting powerful and potent energies for meeting your fitness goals. You can also eliminate information and patterns that keep you unhappy and unhealthy. You will only have to learn a few simple steps to apply this mystical yet practical knowledge for creating your perfect body.

The Colors of the Miraculous

There are hundreds of chakras and even more energy bodies. Fortunately, you can energetically attract your perfect body working with only the main eleven chakras. Figuring out which of your major chakras are strongest and weakest is the key to unfolding and maintaining your perfect body.

The word *chakra* means "spinning wheel of light," and in fact chakras look and work like whirling lights. Seven of the major chakras are based in your spine and specific endocrine glands. Front and back, these chakras spin outward from your body. The remaining four major chakras are located just outside your body.

Every chakra regulates a certain set of physical, emotional, mental, and spiritual concerns. In general, the lower the chakra is with respect to your body, the lower its vibration. Lower vibratory chakras are most frequently related to everyday physical issues, while higher vibratory chakras direct more spiritual concerns.

Each chakra is paired with an auric field. Auric fields are rainbow-colored bands of energies that wrap around your body. The auric layers screen and filter incoming and outgoing sensory and psychic energies, feeding data into and removing energy from your chakras. You could say that your chakras control your internal self while your auric fields handle your external self, as well as your relationship with the outside world. It is important to understand your auric fields as well as your chakras when considering your fitness. Increasing or decreasing the energies of various auric fields can keep unhealthy energies out and allow good energies in.

Chakras and auric fields are typically described as possessing specific colors. These colors indicate the frequencies that dominate the various chakras, as well as the energies that come in and out of them. You could say that you are "coded for the miraculous" in that you can attract everything that you need through your chakras.

Before birth, your spirit programmed its spiritual truths directly into your chakras. These codes include the scripts needed to assure an optimum life, including your dietary, exercise, behavioral, and personal style needs. Thus through your chakras, your physical body is encrypted for your personal perfection. By following these codes, you will exponentially increase the effectiveness of your fitness actions. You will also instinctively magnetize the people, opportunities, and universal energies needed for health, confidence, and perseverance. You will act and think your way to your perfect body.

Determining Your Perfect Body Plan through Stronger and Weaker Chakras

Not every chakra needs to be fully utilized in order to achieve your spiritual purpose. You have only to follow the wisdom of your strongest and most potent chakras to decipher your perfect body codes. By basing your perfect body plan on your strongest chakra programs, you automatically engage the complementary auric fields that magnetize supportive energies and deflect negative ones.

The main determinant of stronger (or more important) and weaker (or less vital) chakras is spiritual. Certain chakras are more active than others in order to support an individual's destiny. All the chakras need to be healthy and functioning, but some are less important than others in an individual's life. You can support your personal destiny and create your perfect body by responding to the needs of your strongest chakras.

We will be looking at the codes of each chakra in chapter 4. This information is needed to help you develop your *perfect body plan*, the plan that will enable you to attract your perfect body. Before you can create your plan, you should determine your *chakra-based personality blueprint*. The personality blueprint is an outline of your chakras, from strongest to weakest. It highlights your probable spiritual mission and gifts, as well as some of the physical characteristics and needs supporting your destiny. By knowing this information, you can discover how to support your strongest chakras and therefore establish the conditions necessary to attract your perfect body.

Ultimately, your perfect body is a means to an end. Your body is a mode of transportation for your spirit and an expression of your spirit that allows you to connect with the world. By creating and maintaining your perfect body, you are undertaking an essential spiritual endeavor. You are agreeing to live as the spirit that you are.

Quiz: Your Strongest Chakras

There are many tests and techniques available for determining your body type, nutritional needs, or exercise requirements. This quiz is different, however, because it aims at pinpointing the underlying spiritual nature of your body so that you can build a perfect body from a spiritual base. By taking this quiz you will separate your strongest from your weakest chakras, which will later enable you to construct your perfect body plan.

Directions: Circle your replies to the following statements on a scale of 0 to 5. Zero means "I disagree completely," while 5 means "I agree completely." You will score the quiz after taking it. Save the results, because you will be working with them throughout this book.

1	My diet is at its worst when I am worried about finances.	0 1 2 3 4 5
2	I like exercising best if I am dressed for the exercise, such as when wearing the right exercise clothing.	0 1 2 3 4 5
3	I desire a fitness program that brings me closer to God or my spiritual guidance.	0 1 2 3 4 5
4	What is the reason for a body? It is my connection to Nature and the natural world.	0 1 2 3 4 5
5	I usually exercise when I am happiest, and I have a hard time when I am not.	0 1 2 3 4 5
6	I stop eating healthily when thinking about all the tragedies in the world.	0 1 2 3 4 5
7	I best alleviate stress through verbal means, such as by listening to music, reading a book, or writing or talking about the problem.	0 1 2 3 4 5
8	I eliminate stress by dealing with the negative thinking causing the problem.	0 1 2 3 4 5
9	I free myself from stress by connecting with family or a loved one.	0 1 2 3 4 5
10	What is the reason for a body? It is a medium for learning and communicating.	0 1 2 3 4 5
11	I like exercises that help me feel able to command superpowers when I am doing them.	0 1 2 3 4 5

12	My diet gets out of control when I am unable to maintain my regular schedule.	0 1 2 3 4 5
13	My ideal fitness program would leave me looking my absolute best to the outside world.	0 1 2 3 4 5
14	It is impossible for me to eat healthy if I am overwhelmed with negativity or feelings of powerlessness.	0 1 2 3 4 5
15	I love any type of exercise or movement—just don't make me sit still for long!	0 1 2 3 4 5
16	I like to dress in clothing that has a magical quality.	0 1 2 3 4 5
17	I cope with stress by tapping into worlds, guides, or powers that are beyond this one.	0 1 2 3 4 5
18	What is the reason for a body? Through it, I connect with others in relationship.	0 1 2 3 4 5
19	I eat an unhealthy diet when I am feeling very emotional.	0 1 2 3 4 5
20	I stop eating a healthy diet when life loses its mysterious, magical quality.	0 1 2 3 4 5
21	I like clothing that shows my personal and spiritual values.	0 1 2 3 4 5
22	My favorite forms of exercise take me outdoors.	0 1 2 3 4 5
23	I like clothing that is intelligent and fit for all the tasks that I have to do on a particular day.	0 1 2 3 4 5
24	What is the reason for a body? It is a crossing point between dimensions and spaces.	0 1 2 3 4 5
25	Relationship problems are my main cause of unhealthy eating.	0 1 2 3 4 5
26	I select clothing that helps me look and feel successful.	0 1 2 3 4 5
27	I forget my stress by helping others with problems more serious than my own.	0 1 2 3 4 5
28	I want a fitness program that incorporates music or learning, such as being taught by a trainer.	0 1 2 3 4 5
29	The optimum fitness program will empower me to be a strong and forceful leader.	0 1 2 3 4 5
30	What is the reason for a body? It is what I inhabit to help change the problems in the world.	0 1 2 3 4 5

31	The ideal fitness program would bring me outdoors and in communion with Nature.	0 1 2 3 4 5
32	It is easiest for me to exercise listening to music, television, or books on tape.	0 1 2 3 4 5
33	A fitness program needs to leave me feeling happier and less emotional.	0 1 2 3 4 5
34	What is the reason for a body? It is who I am. I am my body.	0 1 2 3 4 5
35	What is the reason for a body? It is the vehicle for God and acts of goodness.	0 1 2 3 4 5
36	I like dressing to make a point about a global issue or concern.	0 1 2 3 4 5
37	I like exercise routines, especially if I know which exercises provide which benefits.	0 1 2 3 4 5
38	An ideal fitness program would involve other people, with whom I would become friends through the process.	0 1 2 3 4 5
39	I choose clothes that express my creativity.	0 1 2 3 4 5
40	What is the reason for a body? It is a creative outlet for my inner feelings.	0 1 2 3 4 5
41	What is the reason for a body? It is a command center for powers and forces.	0 1 2 3 4 5
42	I relieve stress by communing with Nature.	0 1 2 3 4 5
43	I eat poorly when my self-image is low.	0 1 2 3 4 5
44	An ideal fitness program would open me to supernatural powers or life's greater mysteries.	0 1 2 3 4 5
45	I do not always pay attention to my clothes; sometimes I am more interested in what I am learning or communicating.	0 1 2 3 4 5
46	I eat an unhealthy diet when I am unable to express my needs or opinions.	0 1 2 3 4 5
47	I work best with stress by praying or meditating as a means of obtaining God's help.	0 1 2 3 4 5
48	I do not eat well when I am stuck indoors and cannot go outside.	0 1 2 3 4 5
49	To alleviate stress, I work. Hard.	0 1 2 3 4 5

50	I like clothing that helps others find me approachable and welcoming.	0 1 2 3 4 5
51	My perfect fitness program would somehow benefit the world, or at least bring its peoples closer together.	0 1 2 3 4 5
52	My stress is alleviated when I am able to forcefully effect change in my life, or in someone else's.	0 1 2 3 4 5
53	I like exercises that put me in touch with supernatural energies or phenomena.	0 1 2 3 4 5
54	What is the reason for a body? It is the visual expression of my inner self.	0 1 2 3 4 5
55	To eliminate stress I have to deal with my feelings.	0 1 2 3 4 5
56	Exercise is easiest if I am praying or meditating.	0 1 2 3 4 5
57	I do not feed myself well if I think I have done something bad or unethical.	0 1 2 3 4 5
58	A good fitness program will clear my mind so I can stay organized and focused.	0 1 2 3 4 5
59	I believe that clothing reflects someone's true personality, so I care about how I look—period.	0 1 2 3 4 5
60	My main goal in a fitness program is to have the energy I must have to be successful, such as in work, primary relationships, sex, and finances.	0 1 2 3 4 5
61	I like clothing that makes me look and feel like a powerful, take-charge leader.	0 1 2 3 4 5
62	I like exercising best with other people.	0 1 2 3 4 5
63	I like types of exercise that teach specific cultural or spiritual concepts.	0 1 2 3 4 5
64	I deal with stress visually, such as by changing clothes or shopping.	0 1 2 3 4 5
65	What is the reason for a body? It holds my thoughts and mind.	0 1 2 3 4 5
66	I only like organic or natural clothing.	0 1 2 3 4 5

Scoring: Add your scores in each of the eleven categories. You will work with the final numbers in the next chapters.

Category One:
1, 15, 26, 34, 49, 60

Category Two:
5, 19, 33, 39, 40, 55

Category Three:
8, 12, 23, 37, 58, 65

Category Four:
9, 18, 25, 38, 50, 62

Category Five:
7, 10, 28, 32, 45, 46

Category Six:
2, 13, 43, 54, 59, 64

Category Seven:
3, 21, 35, 47, 56, 57

Category Eight:
16, 17, 20, 24, 44, 53

Category Nine:
6, 27, 30, 36, 51, 63

Category Ten:
4, 22, 31, 42, 48, 66

Category Eleven:
11, 14, 29, 41, 52, 61

Deciphering Your Personality Blueprint

Magic came where I would, she already knew that. Who knew what she could be if she put her mind to it?

Caitlin Brenna, *The Mountain's Call*

Some of your chakras are stronger than others for an important reason. Your strong chakras contain the gifts that you need in order to achieve your spiritual destiny. They also hold the embryo of your perfect body, the codes that will tell your physical genes, energetic centers, feelings, and mind how to operate in order to shift your perfect body from your hidden depths to concrete reality.

We are going to review the quiz "Your Strongest Chakras" to identify your strongest and weakest chakras. This is to determine your *chakra-based personality blueprint.* The information in this assessment is fundamental for constructing your perfect body program, which will be your action plan for attracting your perfect body.

Your chakra-based personality blueprint highlights your chakras, from strongest to weakest, with respect to your spiritual mission, your spiritual gifts, and the basic physical makeup that supports your destiny. As you activate your strongest chakras in the ways described in this book, you will actually awaken the various traits of your perfect body. As you meet the needs of your strongest chakras, you automatically encourage the healthy behaviors and attitudes that support a perfect body. In addition, as you embrace the spiritual purpose embedded throughout your chakra system, you will attract the magnificence of the universe in support of your total health and happiness.

Now let us look at the lineup of your strongest chakras. Once you have configured this list, you will be ready to develop your perfect body plan—and your own perfect body!

YOUR PERSONALITY BLUEPRINT: YOUR INNERMOST NATURE AND OUTERMOST NEEDS

Most people have one to three strong chakras, but this is not always the case. Some have five or six equally strong chakras, and others' chakras all receive middle-range scores. There is no "right" or "wrong" score, only the score that is right for you.

Your strong chakras are encoded with your strongest spiritual gifts and abilities, as well as the programs for your perfect body and its attributes and needs. You can determine your personality blueprint and therefore perfect body blueprint by arranging your scores to the quiz above.

When scoring the quiz at the end of the previous chapter, you added numbers according to the category of each question. The number of each category is also a number of a chakra. Category one, for example, corresponds with chakra one and category two with chakra two. Each chakra is also paired with an auric field; category one, therefore, corresponds not only to the first chakra, but also to the first auric field, and so on. You will now use these numbers to determine the strength of each of your chakras. You can discover your personality blueprint by ordering the categories and their corresponding chakras from highest to lowest. The highest possible score is 30 and the lowest is 0. You will put tying scores next to each other.

My scores, for instance, look like this:

Category One:	30
Category Two:	16
Category Three:	17
Category Four:	16
Category Five:	28
Category Six:	28
Category Seven:	6
Category Eight:	30
Category Nine:	4
Category Ten:	14
Category Eleven:	21

To obtain my complete personality blueprint, I fill in this box:

Chakra Order Table

Place	Score	Category/Chakra

This is an example of my own chakra order table.

Gift Order Table

Place	Score	Category/Chakra
First place	30 points	1, 8
Second place	28 points	5, 6
Third place	21 points	11
Fourth place	17 points	3
Fifth place	16 points	2, 4
Sixth place	14 points	10
Seventh place	6 points	7
Eighth place	4 points	9

Review your table. Have you accounted for each of the eleven categories, each representing a different chakra and auric field? Now you are ready to begin analyzing your scores to get a glimpse into your personality. Here is an overview of what each chakra means in relation to your spiritual self and, consequently, your body personality.

The Basic Chakra Styles

Chakra One........ Manifester	Chakra Seven..... Spiritualist
Chakra Two........ Feeler	Chakra Eight ...... Shaman
Chakra Three...... Thinker	Chakra Nine .... Idealist
Chakra Four .... Relater	Chakra Ten .... Naturalist
Chakra Five .... Communicator	Chakra Eleven .... Commander
Chakra Six .... Visionary	

Following is a description of each of these eleven basic chakra styles. Review these so that you can start observing your inner nature and body personality through an energetic lens. Each chakra is labeled with a chakra color. Chakras are usually illustrated with specific colors that signify their energetic frequencies. The lower a chakra in relation to the body, the closer it is to infrared hues. Also illustrated is the auric field corresponding to each chakra in terms of your personality and perfect body, so you can begin to work with the amazing properties of these energy bodies. Chakras carry your spiritual and perfect body codes, and your auric fields radiate this information into the world, attracting universal energies to you.

Mentioned as well is the development progression of each chakra. This information tells you when the chakras awaken for the first time in your body. Problems with your chakras and therefore the realization of your perfect body often correlate with difficulties that were incurred when a specific chakra should have opened. If you release the block that manifested in a chakra at a certain age, perhaps because of a traumatic experience, you unlock the codes for your perfect body and attract the energies that you will need in order to build and sustain your perfect body.

Chakra One: Manifester

If anyone loves the physical body and the physical world, it is you. You are the most primal and physical of all the chakra types. Why lie down if you can sit, sit if you can stand, or stand if you can run? This is your attitude in the world, as well. You see a challenge and you are not satisfied until you meet it. Drawn to material reality, you apply your intense and attuned physical resources and strengths to make money, build an empire, have great sex with an equally physically oriented life partner, and move with ease in the world. You are your body and your body is you; therefore, your perfect body assures you complete freedom, connects you in relationship, and is your transportation for success.

Chakra color: Your color is *red*, representing power of movement and passion for life.

First auric field: Your first auric layer releases physical toxins and stress and attracts spiritual energy, which you convert to chemicals and raw energy to drive yourself toward success and pleasure.

Chakra development: This chakra activates in utero until six months of age. You are therefore most affected by issues of safety, security, and worthiness.

Chakra Two: Feeler

Feelings express your soul and connect your soul to your body. To you, every feeling is a unique universe, a mystery to explore, and an adventure in taste and texture. Feelings are the basis of your intense creative abilities, which you offer as your spiritual gift to the universe.

Everything about your body is affected by your feelings and those of others. If you are happy, you will like your body. If you are unhappy, you will not. If you or a loved one is upset, it might be hard for you to eat—or to stop eating! Your body is a holographic representation of how you feel about yourself and what is important to you; therefore, your perfect body is a conduit for emotional and creative expression. You are highly sensual, sensitive, and creative in nature, and you find that everything physical stimulates a distinct emotional reaction. What you eat, how you exercise, and even what you wear consistently needs to keep you emotionally balanced and creatively attuned or your health will suffer for it.

Chakra color: Your color is *orange*, which stimulates feelings, compassion, and innovative expression.

Second auric field: Your second auric field screens out negative feelings, shares positive feelings, and attracts others' feeling energies to you.

Chakra development: The second chakra opens between age six months and two and a half years. At this age, you are strongly influenced by others' moods. Discordance can affect your ability to eat in a healthy manner, exercise, or feel good about your body at this and later ages.

Chakra Three: Thinker

You are best described with a single word: mindful. Information, data, and details fill your fantasies, and you are compelled to organize these bits and pieces of the world into streamlined systems. You are "mindful," meaning you "mind" what your mind needs "to be full of." Your body is therefore extremely affected by the information that you feed it, as well as your ideas about food, exercise, health, and fitness. Your perfect body will enable your brain to function at its best, and allow you to remain focused as you go about organizing the universe, or at least your little pocket of it.

Chakra color: Your color is *yellow*, which reflects the joy of using information in a way that is logical and purposeful.

Third auric field: The third auric layer filters out unhealthy and incorrect psychic and sensory data, so you only acquire healthy and accurate information.

Chakra development: This chakra begins developing between ages two and a half and four and a half years. These years of power struggle affect self-esteem, self-confidence, and later success in the external world. Resultant internal beliefs and external actions establish lifelong patterns that are either physically healthy or unhealthy.

Chakra Four: Relater

You are the heart of the chakra system, attuned to matters of love, healing, and relationship. If your relationships are harmonious you will be happy and hearty. When you experience significant romantic, familial, work, or friendship-based problems, your physical health becomes compromised. As a healer, you have the capacity to help heal yourself or others in difficult times, but you have to establish good boundaries or you will lose your own vital energy and develop bodily problems.

Chakra color: Your color is *green*, signifying the power to heal and change.

Fourth auric field: The fourth layer attracts healing energies and healthy relationships while deflecting harmful energies. Essentially, it assures the giving and receiving of love.

Chakra development: The fourth chakra is stimulated between the ages of four and a half and six and a half, key years for developing authentic relationships with family and peers. Lack of self-acceptance, rejection from others, abandonment from a parent, and other wounds involving relationship and love can cause a lack of self-love, and therefore problems in taking care of your own health.

Chakra Five: Communicator

Communicators are about learning, teaching, educating, and listening, and when that is all done, they start the communication process all over again. A pure Communicator will be physically healthy if allowed to share and learn.

Chakra color: Your color is *blue*, which reflects the giving and receiving of information for higher ends.

Fifth auric field: The fifth auric field sorts verbal data, opening you to higher wisdom and guidance and filtering harmful or inapplicable auditory information.

Chakra development: The fifth chakra is activated from ages six and a half to eight and a half, greatly increasing a child's potential for accessing higher information and guidance. Messages that compromise your ability to receive, share, or exchange personal or learned information can shut down this chakra and, therefore, stifle spiritual development and physical health.

Chakra Six: Visionary

True Visionaries live up to the name. They are futuristic, strategic, and, above all, imaginative. Your spiritual pursuits will always involve long-term plans aimed at meeting long-range goals. Visual by nature, you will be highly attentive to your appearance.

Chakra color: Your color is *purple*, which symbolizes majesty and magic. What's the root of both words? *Mage.* Visionaries are mages who peer into the future to make practical, here-and-now decisions.

Sixth auric field: This field snares potential futures and enables you to project them forward in your mind's eye. Upon seeing what is possible, you can then decide what is practical to do today.

Chakra development: The sixth chakra awakens during ages eight and a half through thirteen. This period involves the development of the self-image, which is greatly affected by internalized projections from family, society, and the culture at large. All these players and your reactions to them factor into your body image, which affects every aspect of your physical well-being.

Chakra Seven: Spiritualist

If you are a Spiritualist, you are here to spread divinity. Your body is therefore a means of serving a greater power. If you believe that your body is good, you will be in good health; if you think it is bad, your health will suffer.

Chakra color: Your color is *white*, a color that illuminates spiritual truths. In the Western world, white represents purity, sanctity, honesty, integrity, and spirituality, all of which are indicative of a Spiritualist's grounding values, which serve as fodder for his or her spiritual purpose.

Seventh auric field: The seventh auric layer is an access point to spiritual realms, spirits and ghosts, and energies of the Divine. Good health depends upon allowing in energies that match your personal spirit.

Chakra development: The seventh chakra unlocks between ages fourteen and twenty-one, opening spiritual energies to help you heal from life's wounds and attract what you need in order to achieve your destiny.

Chakra Eight: Shaman

Shamans experience life inside out, upside down, and turned around. They are therefore considered life's masters of mystery, able to perceive what others cannot. Able to link worlds and dimensions, they unify nature, humankind, and the worlds of spirits, and their purpose always involves using these connections for healing self and others. Shamans often utilize their bodies as conduits for healing or supernatural energies, and their health is therefore either adversely or positively affected by the rituals they use for their work.

Chakra color: Your color is *black* or *silver*. Black represents the mystery of using negativity for positive reasons, while silver symbolizes the purity of providing information for the greater good.

Eighth auric field: The eighth auric field links all dimensions, planes, and time periods into a center point. It then filters energies or entities that are needed from those that are unnecessary or harmful.

Chakra development: The eighth chakra opens between ages twenty-one and twenty-eight, triggering issues from your past and encouraging the development of potent magical gifts.

Chakra Nine: Idealist

Idealists are the world's harmonizers, desiring communion among people everywhere. As an Idealist, you can peer into the heart of a matter or the soul of a person and initiate action that can blend heart and soul. Your physical health will therefore be affected by the causes you pursue, and your ability to take care of yourself while taking care of others.

Chakra color: Your color is *gold*. Gold magnetizes love, infusing people and situations with grace and goodness.

Ninth auric field: The ninth field initiates contact with higher-order beings, including masters, avatars, and saints, drawing on entities and individuals that are supportive of humanity's continual development. Physically, it allows penetration of ideas or universal energies that attune the individual to the collective whole, and it rejects energies that might harm the individual or a larger group.

Chakra development: The ninth chakra is first activated during preconception, selecting physical genes supportive of your soul purpose and life mission. It again rouses between ages twenty-eight and thirty-five, linking individuals to their soul purpose and spiritual helpers.

Chakra Ten: Naturalist

It is easy to spot a Naturalist. They are the people with Birkenstock sandals, organic cotton underwear, and sprouts on their sandwiches. Naturalists find paradise in the world of Nature, preferring the great outdoors to the narrow confines of cement cities. A Naturalist's spiritual mission is always linked to the benefit of the environment, the home, or the wellness of natural beings. Attuned to Nature, a Naturalist is dependent upon his or her natural surroundings for physical health.

Chakra color: Your color is *brown*, signifying all things natural.

Tenth auric field: The tenth field surrounds the skin and holds the programs for your perfect body, as regulated by your spirit.

Chakra development: During preconception the tenth chakra works with the ninth to select physical genetics to match your soul purpose. It then reengages between ages thirty-five and forty-two to help you ground your purpose in practical reality.

Chakra Eleven: Commander

You are a natural-born leader, ready to access your vast resources and powerful personality to change the world. Like the Shaman, you can summon potent powers and forces from the worlds of humanity or Nature to meet your goals. Do you want to quench a fire? Depending upon your training and skill, you might call a waterfall to meet your demands—or a troop of firefighters. Your physical health will depend upon the appropriate and ethical use of your powers and abilities, as well as your skill at transforming negative into positive energy.

Chakra color: Your color is *rose,* combining the red of passion with the spirituality of white to create loving power.

Eleventh auric field: This field encompasses the entire body, concentrating in the hands and the feet, which serve as command centers for natural and supernatural energies.

Chakra development: The eleventh chakra engages between the ages of forty-two and forty-nine, encouraging the full expression of your personal powers and leadership to effect world change.

ASSESSING YOUR INNER NATURE: YOUR PERSONALITY BLUEPRINT SCORES

We will now review your quiz scores and compare them with the primary eleven chakra types to illustrate your inner nature. This information will later help you determine your perfect body blueprint.

Fill in the following table to outline your chakra strengths.

Chakra Personality Table

Place	Score	Title/s

This is an example of my own chakra personality table.

My Chakra Personality Table

Place	Score	Title/s
First place	30 points	Manifester Shaman
Second place	28 points	Communicator Visionary
Third place	21 points	Commander
Fourth place	17 points	Thinker
Fifth place	16 points	Feeler Relater
Sixth place	14 points	Naturalist
Seventh place	6 points	Spiritualist
Eighth place	4 points	Idealist

You have just outlined your *chakra personality order*, listing your personalities from strongest to weakest. It will be easier to work with this information by summarizing it further, according to these three categories:

- Strong
- Supportive
- Weak

Your highest scores indicate your strong chakras. These chakras hold your most crucial spiritual attributes and reflect your most necessary physical traits, drives, and needs. These chakras and their corresponding auric fields can be vitalized to attract energies for perfecting your body. Supportive chakras—those with scores that fall in the midrange—are less developed and, therefore, less critical than your strong chakras, but they are still important to your overall well-being. They can sustain your strong chakras when you are under pressure, and take over physical processes when strong chakra physical functions wane or fail. Your weak chakras are your lowest-scoring chakras. Usually, they represent attributes and abilities that are unimportant to your spiritual mission. Sometimes these are wounded or injured chakras, holding repressed feelings or issues. If this is the case, it is imperative to work on these chakra issues therapeutically or medically.

Your strong chakras are those that score 23 or higher or are your own highest-scoring chakras. Supportive chakras typically score between 14 and 22 and fall mid-range in your chart. Weak chakras are those that score between 0 and 13, or hug the bottom of your scores. Generally, your most important scores are your top three and your very lowest. These indicate your greatest attributes and your "don't even try" traits. Knowing your supportive chakras tells you what strengths you can draw upon when stressed or when you need to compensate for weaknesses.

The following will help you further understand your personality profile.

1. *If you have one strong chakra*... Your spiritual mission and therefore your personality are largely based in one chakra, the strength of which is indomitable. You will show certainty of thought and action if fully utilizing this gift, and you will be firm about the type of diet, exercise, and health care that suit your needs. Be careful, though. It is easy to burn out a single chakra, as well as your physical body, if you push too hard. Supplement your professional and personal life with encouragement from your supportive chakras to assure physical and psychological health.

2. *If you have two strong chakras*... You reveal two strong aptitudes to the world. If these are complementary, your career, relationships, and health care will seem relatively easy and simple. Sometimes our strong chakras seem oppositional, which challenges us to incorporate all components of our personality. Seek to enfold

your two strong chakras and meet their physical needs by thinking creatively, without limitations.

3. *If you have three strong chakras . . .* Having multiple gifts and talents can be either fun and enriching—or challenging and confusing. It inspires the question of what, how, and when to eat, exercise, or perform other mandatory physical tasks. Which self wins out in the debate? I encourage three-chakra persons to imagine a triangle and attach a chakra type to each of its corners. Now decide which set of attributes to assert as primary in different situations. This way you transform your other two strong chakras into supportive chakras. You do not lose their power; neither do you establish the ground for conflict.

4. *If you have four strong chakras . . .* Which self do you want to be today? That might be the most pressing question in your mind when you arise. Your varying abilities and strengths can create tension within yourself or with others, as you adapt according to your situation and your needs. Diverse health care practices will support your perfect body. I suggest that four-chakra people picture their gifts as forming the four corners of a square. Squares represent stability. Allow each gift to influence every decision. This way you create a unified whole and internal well-being.

5. *If you have more than four strong chakras . . .* On one hand, you are extremely gifted and well-rounded. On the other hand, you have so many different qualities that you are probably overwhelmed! Internal tension between your various chakras can lead to depression or anxiety. Judgments from others who want you to choose who or what to be can ironically cause low self-esteem and a poor body image. Learn about boundaries. Train yourself to set specific goals and establish the parameters that you need in order to keep your energy controlled and in focus. Think of what you could accomplish if all your strengths were pulling together instead of pulling you apart!

6. *If your chakras are primarily in the mid-range . . .* In all likelihood, you were popular and well liked at school. It is easy for you to be accepted and be what others want you to be. Social skills aside, there is probably more to you than you are letting others—or yourself—see. Almost everyone has at least one strong chakra. If it is not apparent, there is a reason that it has been hidden. Sometimes the causes are familial judgments, religious opinions, or cultural prejudices. Unearth the reason that you felt—or feel—safer hiding your powerful self and obtain the support you need in order to unfold your true self in the world.

7. *If you have many weak chakras . . .* In a world that defends perfectionism, it is important to hear a contrary message. There is nothing wrong with having many weaknesses! You cannot be perfect at everything. It is more important to excel at what you can be excellent at than to waste energy trying to achieve the unattainable. Having many weak chakras and no strong chakras, however, *is* a warning sign. If you are also lacking in physical strength or stamina, signs that you are hiding behind your weaknesses rather than living from your strengths, it is especially important that you heed the warning. Somewhere along the line you might have decided that it was unsafe to show your greatness. What were you good at when you were young? What did you want to be when you grew up? I encourage you to explore these issues with a professional therapist or spiritual guide if you think that you have unseen abilities.

Printing Out a Blueprint: Developing Your Personality Profile

It is time to begin putting together the puzzle pieces of your personality. This exercise will help you assemble a picture of your true personality. You can also use this process to assist someone else in putting together his or her own personality blueprint.

Complete these statements for yourself or someone else:

• These are my strongest chakras and related character traits:

- The total of these strongest chakra traits means that I am interested in the following:
- And that I will usually act like this:
- And that I will want the following out of life:
- And that I will have the following types of physical or bodily needs and desires:
- Based on my strengths, I would suggest that my spiritual purpose involves the following:
- These are my supportive chakras and corresponding character traits:
- These supportive chakra traits mean that I am interested in the following:
- And that I can draw on these characteristics to assist myself under pressure:
- And that I can do the following to compensate for weaknesses:
- And that I can do the following to support my spiritual destiny:
- These are my weak chakras and corresponding chakra deficiencies:
- These weak chakras mean that I will lack the ability or drive to:
- And that I will not be interested in:
- And that I will be vulnerable to:
- And that I will lack the physical capacity for:
- And that I must do the following to compensate:
- In three sentences, I would now describe myself like this:

A Narrative on the Self

In the previous exercise you completed statements that helped you reflect upon your chakra-based personality. I now encourage you to write a narrative about yourself (or the person you assessed). Describing your personality in a narrative is a great way to fully embrace all aspects of your personality without judgment. Self-acceptance is the basis for attracting and accepting your perfect body.

Some people do not like analyzing themselves. You might feel self-conscious, as if you are bragging, or conversely you might feel bad about yourself. You might wonder how you can be objective when you are the subject. Self-analysis, however, is an objective process when you use the chakras as its basis. Use their truth to seek deeper truths and you will be surprised at what you will learn about yourself.

As an example, I am going to analyze my own chakra personality in a narrative format. I recommend writing about yourself in the third person to help reduce self-consciousness and increase objectivity.

Cyndi has four strong chakras, which means that she has multiple gifts and must address the stresses that accompany this profile. Her top scores are close to one another and indicate she is a Manifester, Shaman, Communicator, and Visionary. Combined, these attributes mark her as an extremely forceful person with a high drive for material success. She is able to access the gifts of communicating and strategizing to encourage shamanic changes for herself and others. Physically, she must maintain her physical strength to serve as the shamanic portal between worlds; conversely, her health will suffer if she is unable to use her visual or communication gifts to support this higher cause.

Cyndi has several supportive chakras to assist her in meeting her life mission. As a Shaman, she is most likely to access her secondary Commander gifts to summon otherworldly or even environmental energies for her purpose, and she is able either to hear or to picture these powers through her gifts as a Communicator and Visionary. As a Manifester, she can draw upon her leadership qualities to achieve the worldly success that she desires.

Her other supportive chakras, which lend her abilities in thinking, feeling, and relating, can be extremely useful under stress. As a Thinker, she can use logic to assess situations and strategize for change. By combining her feeling and relating attributes, she can soften her otherwise assertive approach to life and relationships and touch others with compassion and love. When experiencing a crisis, she can refresh herself through connecting to Nature. Though not overly dependent on Mother Nature, her score of 14 indicates that getting outside can be calming.

As for being a Spiritualist or an Idealist, she might as well surrender right now. Her motives for life and health care are not, nor will they ever be, idealistic. With such high scores as a Manifester and a Shaman, her reasons for wanting fitness and style will be self-oriented and a mystery to anyone but herself.

Can you see the benefit of writing your own personality narrative? Don't be shy! Be honest. We all have strengths and weaknesses. That is the reason that we are all on this planet at the same time. Together, we can accomplish quite a lot.

From Destiny to Delivery: What Is the Personality of Your Perfect Body?

"You are old, Father William," the young man said.
"And your hair has become very white;
And yet you incessantly stand on your head—
Do you think, at your age, it is right?"

Lewis Carroll, *Alice's Adventures in Wonderland*

Your Ultimate Body

Your perfect body is already intact. It is the mighty oak nestled inside the acorn. At this moment, perhaps, your perfect body is only a seed of potential, but the tiniest spark of life can grow into the grandest tree in the forest.

The potential for your perfect body is encoded within your chakras, and you can, at any time, transform your current body into its ideal form. Your strongest chakras are the most powerful blueprints of your perfect body. These core chakras, programmed by your spirit, can tell your brain which foods and exercises will encourage perfection. They can instruct your physical organs how to process data, nutrients, and ideas for your well-being. These supervising chakras can also disseminate energies regarding boundaries, emotional needs, and relationship desires into corresponding auric fields, which in turn tell the world how to respond to you. It is one thing to agonize in silence as you refuse a delectable dessert of homemade chocolate cake. How much easier it is to have loved ones "read" the fact that you really want to eat a healthy diet and they serve you salad, sushi, or a bowl of fresh strawberries!

Your perfect body is unique. A friend might need to drink wheatgrass shakes to sculpt the ideal body. You could have a body that thrives on meat and potatoes. As the poem introducing this chapter suggests, one person might need to stand on his head to become his true self, while another is better off learning how to slow dance. By listening to and using the information of your strongest chakras, you can unfold the body that is perfect for you, regardless of your age, gender, ethnicity, background, and income level.

The Personality of Your Body: From Spirit to Body

Chakra personality types will share perfect body traits with one another. There are two main reasons for this. The first is spiritual and the second is biological.

Spiritually, the people that constitute a chakra personality group, such as all Manifesters, will have similar spiritual purposes and gifts. In order to express these spiritual functions, members of a chakra personality group must be biologically able to channel the energies that encourage their primary spiritual mission. Thus, each personality group will have specific physical values, needs, and capabilities. A "perfect body" for a Feeler, then, will intrinsically differ from a "perfect body" for a Thinker. In addition, all Feelers will have some perfect body traits in common, as will all Thinkers.

Most energy workers see chakras as esoteric organs. But chakras control so much more than metaphysical constructs. Because they use both psychic and sensory energies, they manage all aspects of your physical well-being. The easiest way to address the exact biological functions of your chakras is to consider the relationship of the chakras to the endocrine system. By centering certain components of your perfect body plan on your strongest chakra's core endocrine gland, you can intensify the unfolding of your perfect body. Of course, you will want to consider medical factors and input from your doctor, but linking the chakras to the endocrine system with your diet and exercise program is one way to accelerate to tachyon speed!

Chakras and Your Endocrine Glands

Each chakra regulates a different endocrine gland, which is the basis of its distinct role in the body. Every endocrine gland produces a very specific set of hormones, which are chemicals that have a regulatory or stimulatory effect. Hormones enter the bloodstream and cause chain reactions that establish the health of your nervous system, organic functions, emotional state, and all other aspects of the body and your life. Of course, hormones do not work in a vacuum. Endocrine glands respond to any number of other factors, including your emotional state, electromagnetic currents, diet, organic health, muscular strength, memories, attitudes, and much more. Hormones also react to other hormones in a complex fashion.

Categorizing body types and health practices according to the glandular system is not a new concept. Various Eastern medical practices have used this framework for thousands of years. Acupuncture, a form of meridian healing, attributes all medical conditions to an imbalance in chi, the flow of life energy, as regulated by the organs. Thus, a

Chinese medical practitioner might attribute a weight issue to the kidney, liver, or spleen meridian. The East Indian practice of Ayurvedic medicine also considers body types, asserting that there are three basic organ-based body categories. Some Western practitioners are finally considering these organ-based connections. Consider, for example, the work of individuals such as American scientist Roger Williams, who classifies individuals according to three basic types based on the endocrine glands of the adrenals, pituitary, and thyroid. We will draw upon his ideas, which he terms the "genetotrophic concept," when working with the first, fifth, and sixth chakras in particular.[2]

What happens if you link chakras with your endocrine system in pursuit of your perfect body? Let us say that you are primarily a fourth chakra–based person, which means that your major endocrine gland is the heart. The heart generates 50,000 times more femtoteslas—a measure of the electomagnetic field—than does the brain, and more than any other organ in the body. As a heart-based person, you will have a strong electrical system and corresponding personality traits. Issues involving love will affect your physical health. Love will result in a perfect body. Lack of love will cause a crisis in the electrical system and related health challenges.

Here is a description of the chakras as they relate to the endocrine system, as I have determined through research and my own work.

Chakra	Physical Location	Endocrine Glands or Related System
First	Groin or genital area	Adrenals
Second	Abdomen	Ovaries in women and testes in men
Third	Solar plexus	Pancreas
Fourth	Chest	Heart
Fifth	Throat	Thyroid
Sixth	Forehead	Pituitary
Seventh	Top of the head	Pineal
Eighth	An inch above the head	Thymus
Ninth	A foot above the head	Diaphragm
Tenth	A foot under the feet	Bone marrow
Eleventh	Around the body	Connective tissue; strongest around hands and feet

No chakra group can be termed healthy or unhealthy. Neither is there a good or bad perfect body. There is only *your* perfect body, which you already inhabit, whether or not it is apparent in the mirror.

CUSTOMIZING YOUR BODY

Let us look at the eleven major personality types through the filter of the physical body and its needs. This way, you can become familiar with the means for unlocking your perfect body and habits that will attract energies to create and sustain it. I will be examining each chakra type in relation to the following characteristics, to help you begin constructing your final perfect body plan.

- Spiritual Motivation
- Endocrine Effects
- Diet
- Exercise
- Pitfalls and False Pleasures
- Success Tips
- Style
- Supportive Assistants

Chakra One: Manifester

Spiritual Motivation: You are determined to manifest your spiritual truths and energies in physical form. Ultimately, you perfect your body to achieve material success, which you deem to be as worthy an endeavor as striving for spiritual peace.

Endocrine Effects: Manifesters express themselves through their adrenal glands, miniature organs that sit atop the kidneys. The adrenals are the stress organs of the body, emitting hormones like adrenaline, hydrocortisol, and cortisol, all of which pump you up and cool you down under pressure. If your adrenals are kept healthy and happy, you will be the physical powerhouse of the chakra system!

Diet: Manifesters require dense yet energizing food to maintain their fast-forward drive. Generally, the first chakra is best sustained by carnivorous eating, unless this is medically inadvisable. Manifesters burn up vast amounts of life energy, and the best physical source for this energy includes animal protein sources. Think "red" and you have described most first chakra foods, which include red meat, tomatoes, beets, and dark berries. Other foods include those produced by animals, such as dairy products.

Exercise: Even asleep, a Manifester is ready to pounce on tomorrow's opportunities. Because of the immense pressure that a Manifester puts upon him- or herself to achieve, exercise is necessary to relieve stress.

I recommend that Manifesters select at least one of these three exercises for discipline and self-control.

- Martial arts to blend spiritual qualities with physical exercise while encouraging muscular discipline.
- Walking to calm and soothe the mind and the muscles, both of which tense in reaction to the Manifester's fast-paced lifestyle.
- Weight lifting to train a Manifester's sometimes-brutal power.

A Manifester must also select a complete and intense aerobic exercise to release adrenal stress hormones; one possibility is brisk walking. Many Manifesters, however, select more daredevil disciplines, such as downhill skiing, mountain biking, swimming, running, rock climbing, and other ambitious, full-body activities.

Pitfalls and False Pleasures: There are two primary problem areas for those of us who have a strong first chakra. Some Manifesters overestimate their physical prowess and push to the point of hurting their bodies. Others tire of striving and simply give up. Here are some warning signs that you are nearing either side of the continuum.

- Wear and tear on the physical body. Especially watch out for your joints, bones, and muscles.
- Burned-out adrenals. If you push yourself to the edge, you can stretch too far and fall! Warning signs of burned-out adrenals include fatigue, exhaustion, depression, and circulation issues; sensitivities to meat, sugars, carbohydrates, and dairy products; and

reactivity to substances like bacterial toxins, histamine, drugs, poisons, and hormones, including insulin and thyroxin.

- Workaholism. The enthused Manifester is on a one-way road to success. If financial or career success is the only goal, then everything and everyone else will be low priority in the Manifester's life.

- Sex addiction or sexual fears. The healthy first-chakra person loves sex, an outgrowth of a passionate nature. Sexual fears and sex addiction have as their common root an avoidance of intimacy.

- Overindulgence. Life is to be tasted, says the extreme Manifester, who can be found gorging on life's luxuries, including fine wines, chocolates, foods, sexual games, and expensive play items.

- Addictions. Manifesters' main life issues include learning how to manage their primal feelings and urges. Failure to cope with these internal drives can lead to alcoholism, anorexia, bulimia, or obesity, as well as workaholism, shopaholism, gambling, and narcotic addictions.

- Issues of shame and low sense of self-worth. Manifesters' personal challenges often stem from their belief that they are worthless. This deep-seated problem often originates in chakra-based issues that occur in utero and up to six months of age; from early childhood abuse; or from significant life challenges, such as severe poverty, rape, religious brainwashing, or parental addictions.

- Abusiveness or victimization. When their self-worth is compromised, some Manifesters become abusive, dominating others to feel more powerful. Others, most often women, might play the role of the victim, sublimating their own desires to avoid internal rage and pain.

- Erosion of health. Manifesters can fall prey to physical challenges, such as low metabolism and therefore weight issues, constant infections, blood and circulation issues, kidney problems (which can lead to diabetes or heart disease), chronic fatigue and exhaustion, and early aging. In addition, there is a correlation between reduced adrenal function and the incidence of asthma.

Success Tips: In a word, adapt! You feel powerful and dynamic and you tend to force things, confident that your approach will achieve what you want. It might serve you better at times, however, to be less forceful.

- Eat three meals a day, and emphasize protein.
- Eat a modest amount of carbohydrates, and consider restricting your consumption of dairy, sugars, yeast, alcohol, fruits, and most bread products.
- Supplement with stress vitamins, including vitamins C and B; in particular, take extra B_5 for your adrenals. Take zinc with your B vitamins. Consider a liquid mineral supplement.
- Drink ten to fifteen glasses of water a day, which is necessary for adrenal support.
- Sleep at least seven or eight hours a night. You have earned it.
- Meditate or pray. Learn active meditation, which involves breathing deeply and clearing the mind while exercising, doing housework, washing the car, or performing any other activity.
- Try a competitive sport. Most participants in competitive sports are Manifesters. A Manifester thrives on competition.
- Take up golf or any other hard-driving sport that appeals to your competitive edge. I suspect that the majority of golfers are highly driven Manifesters, seeking success while getting in their exercise. Tennis, racquetball, and many other group sports are also excellent for conducting business while playing.
- Schedule time for loved ones, play, and recreation. Manifesters tend to let work take over their lives.
- Take many vacations, especially if they are adventure trips. Moreover, turn off the cell phone.
- Bodywork. Try massage, acupuncture, or chiropractic arts.
- Love your job and your primary life partner. If these two areas make you unhappy, you will become grumpy, unpleasant, addictive, and unhealthy.
- See a therapist. If you experience shame operating in your life, obtain professional help.

Style: The Manifester dresses for success in a chosen industry. If you want to climb the corporate ladder to the top, you will dress like a

CEO when you are still in the mailroom—and you will be the best-dressed CEO once you ascend to the height of your career.

Supportive Assistants:
- A personal trainer. Manifesters excel under tutelage.
- An accountability coach. Instead of joining a support group, hire a personal coach who emphasizes goals and concrete successes. Make health a job and you will achieve it!
- An expert shopper. You know how to dress for success but probably don't have the time to do the shopping.
- A chef, a favorite restaurant, a good fast-food place, or a life partner who likes to cook. Most Manifesters do not have a lot of extra time. If you want to eat healthy, arrange for someone else to cook!
- An aesthetician or a dermatologist. The first auric field includes the skin. Keeping your skin healthy infuses health into your body and soul.
- A therapist. If you are feeling or exhibiting signs of emotional distress, seek professional help. Move from striving to thriving.
- A professional body worker. Massage will help release stress held in the body.
- Heroes and mentors, alive, deceased, or legendary. Only a lucky few Manifesters find live mentors who can guide them into the unknown. If you cannot find a suitable mentor, follow an idea suggested by Napoleon Hill in his book *Think and Grow Rich* (Ballantine Books). Create a board of directors of admirable heroes in your imagination, and consult them in your mind when you need insight.

Chakra Two: Feeler

Spiritual Motivation: Ultimately, your spiritual purpose involves expressing your feelings through creative means. If you repress or deny your feelings, you will become angry and overeat out of spite. If you have become a caretaker of others' feelings, you become depressed and overweight. Color your world with harmonious feelings and the world will become the colorful place it was meant to be for you.

Endocrine Effects: The endocrine glands for female Feelers are their ovaries; for men, it is their testes. Energetically, these organs convert spiritual forces, which include feelings, into organic chemicals. Physically, these glands work in cooperation with the hypothalamus, which is a gland in the brain, to produce peptide chains (or proteins) that send feelings throughout the body. If you hold happy and positive beliefs, your hypothalamus cascades your body with peptide chains that inspire and motivate. If you suffer from unhappy or negative beliefs, your hypothalamus floods you with difficult and life-inhibiting emotions. Developing your perfect body as a Feeler is determined by the feelings or peptide chains that run your life.

Diet: The ovaries produce estrogen and progesterone, while the testes are responsible for testosterone. In general, Feelers should customize their diets in response to their sexual development stage and by eating to moderate their hormones. One application of this advice is age-related. A twenty-year-old male Feeler producing a large amount of testosterone can tolerate more food low in nutritional content than can a fifty-year-old andropausal man with less muscle-producing testosterone. A twenty-year-old female Feeler, at the top of her progesterone and estrogen production, must eat differently than a fifty-year-old Feeler woman going through menopause.

The age and vitality of the sexual glands also affect people actively seeking their perfect bodies. Estrogen is held in fat cells. When women diet, some of this estrogen is released into the circulatory system, throwing off their hormonal balance. This imbalance can lead to depression and often carbohydrate cravings. If a woman's estrogen levels fall, such as before and during menopause, and her testosterone remains at the same level as before menopause, she will experience hair loss. Men might lose hair as their testosterone levels increase or drop in relation to their other hormones as well.

Regardless of gender, Feelers who do not eat according to age and body type are highly susceptible to an infestation of candida, a yeast organism. Candida can proliferate inside the intestines, in the reproductive system, or atop bodily organs. Candida feeds off sugar, therefore causing you to crave sweets to assure a steady stream of their favorite food. As a by-product, they produce substances that clog your immune and lymph systems and prevent healthy cellular metabolism, thereby depriving your cells of nutrition. Candida stimulates you to eat more while starving you to death.

If you are a susceptible Feeler, you might want to prevent or break this candida stranglehold by entirely avoiding sugar, gluten, dairy, and yeast. Opt for second-chakra foods, which include oranges, yams, and salmon; whole grains, including wheat and oats (unless you are sensitive or while infested with candida); and poultry such as chicken and turkey. Select fruit over juices, which increase candida and other acid-producing intestinal growths. Select orange and colored vegetables over white potatoes and root vegetables, because the sugars in the latter promote carbohydrate cravings. Choose hormone-free meat if possible, as you are probably sensitive to chemical preservatives or added animal hormones.

Exercise: Feelers can get lost in the world of feelings and myriad sensual urges. Exercise compensates by clearing emotions and the mind, thus encouraging internal and external forces to perfect the body. I do not know many strong Feelers who like to exercise, preferring the pampering of massage to the toil of physical exercise. Still, it is important to move your body, if only to enjoy the deliciousness of life! Feelers prosper with full-body (and sensuous) sports like tai chi, Pilates, yoga, and dance, or water sports like swimming.

Pitfalls and False Pleasures: Feelings take a toll, as does repressed or overemphasized creativity. Feelers, be alert for these tendencies:

- Gluttony and sloth. You love the pleasures of the body, and if you are particularly bored, you can overindulge. Difficult feelings can help you convince yourself that you really *deserve* that piece of chocolate cake!
- Emotionalism. It is one thing to feel your feelings, but it is another to become your feelings. In general, depression indicates repressed feelings and physical toxicity, while anxiety reveals fears about the future and beliefs in lack and limitation.

- Oversympathizing. Feelers tend to absorb others' feelings. Feelings are made of energy, and energy can be passed from person to person, thus clogging the Feeler's system.
- Hormone imbalance. Because of the Feeler's dependency on basic sexual hormones and peptide chains of feelings, Feelers are highly susceptible to hormone imbalances.
- Codependency. Feelers find it easy to become codependents, taking care of others' feelings while sacrificing their own needs.
- Confusion. To be confused means to be "fused with" something or someone else. This is an energetic condition similar to the psychological state of codependency. You will not develop your perfect body by assuming someone else's identity.
- Creative mania. It is great to love the creative process, but some Feelers lose themselves in art to avoid the pain of feelings.
- Addictions. Feelers are prone to "luxury addictions," such as shopping, overeating, and emotionalism. Substance addictions cause cravings for softer foods, like wheat, yeast, sugar, and dairy products, which provide a false sense of comfort in what can appear to be a difficult world.
- Distorted feelings and beliefs. Most Feelers' mental or emotional disorders stem from issues that arose between the ages of six months and two and a half years, and from relationships that stifle their feelings.
- Physical illnesses. Feelers' illnesses include the already-mentioned candida, as well as fungus and bacteria, all of which grow in an acidic environment; various "itises" like diverticulitis, appendicitis, endometriosis, and irritable bowel syndrome; lower back problems; cancers, growths, and other problems in the uterine, abdominal, or testicular regions, including prostate cancer; and autoimmune and immune disorders.

Success Tips:
- Diet. Test for food sensitivities and allergies, especially for grains, gluten, sugars, yeast, and dairy. Refrain from eating these substances if there is a problem. Use computer-based healing devises like BioSET therapy (see page 136) to clear these allergies. I have

found that many female Feelers, especially those nearing or in menopause, respond well to some of the recommendations made by Dr. Diana Schwarzbein in her book *The Schwarzbein Principles* (HCI).

- Increase your fiber. Fiber prevents colon problems.
- Drink plenty of water. Feelers require at least ten glasses of water a day to flush toxins.
- Take a bath. Soak away stress with Epsom salts and ginger to release others' feelings and your own bottled-up emotions.
- Utilize a medical professional. Watch out for abdominal or reproductive issues. Women, get your Pap smears. Men, check your PSA or prostate numbers. Both sexes, watch for colon cancer and consider hormonal supplementation when Nature calls for it, preferably using natural or bioidentical hormones.
- Supplement for security. Some women benefit from soy supplementation, black cohosh, black currant oil, evening primrose oil, and increased minerals when they are undergoing hormonal changes; I recommend liquid supplement programs. Some natural care physicians also recommend saw palmetto for men (or women) if high testosterone levels or supplements are causing hair loss; saw palmetto also seems to positively impact the prostate.
- Wear bright colors. Wear the colors that bring you joy and happiness. If you are going to be with difficult people, consider wearing black, which repels others' energies.
- Drink red wine, if you can safely consume alcohol. There are dozens of research projects at renowned institutions, including Harvard Medical School, Brown University, the University of Connecticut, and the Fred Hutchinson Cancer Center, asserting the benefits of red wine. Apparently, it contains an ingredient called resveratrol, found to increase the life span of every organism it is given to. Other studies show that red wine reduces the number and size of fat cells in the body, can cut your risks of colon and prostate cancer by 50 percent or more, and provides benefits for the heart.
- Dance. Dancing releases any negative energy from others that you are holding onto.

- Deal with your despair. A study at Yale showed that women were more apt to lose weight and keep it off if they maintained a behavior-oriented program until they actually increased their self-confidence and self-esteem. Believe in yourself and you can do it!
- Practice auric protection. Imagine your second auric field as surrounded by shinglelike mirrors. Program the overall field so that others' energies bounce back to the "higher self" of the sender by visualizing yourself writing a message on this mirror, such as "I only accept energies useful to myself."
- Practice auric attraction. Imagine feeling happy and having already achieved your goals. Imagine writing these accomplishments with a white marker on orange paper. Next, envision yourself pinning these "wishing papers" onto your second auric field. Ask the Divine to infuse these requests with love in order to attract your dreams to you.

Style: A Feeler is always original, emanating sensuality and personality. Feelers wear their personalities on their exterior, and they will be happiest when dressed in clothing that emphasizes their creative nature. Among the chakra types, Feelers are the most attracted to and affected by fragrance and clothing texture, quality, color, and fashion. Select a style based on your creative spirit and you will quickly achieve success!

Supportive Assistants:
- Groups. Feelers love and can greatly benefit from group membership, when they participate in them with healthy boundaries. Overeaters Anonymous, a diet support group, an exercise support group, an intuition development class, a painting club, or a dance class can all help a Feeler achieve the goal of a perfect body.
- Spiritual forces. Various spiritual energies and forces help the Feeler repel or release others' feelings. I recommend using inner vision to wash your internal body with white energy. Visualize a cascade of light water entering through the top of your head and flowing through and around your body. Both physical and psychic

debris is gathered in this stream and absorbed in the earth. You can use this same technique to cleanse with pink or orange colors as well. Pink will suffuse you with love and organize with positive feelings, whereas white is a good general cleanser.

• Spiritual guides. Feelers are tempted to fix everyone else's feelings. Instead, request the Divine to help others—and yourself!

Chakra Three: Thinker

Spiritual Motivation: Thinkers love information. Mental acuity is the cornerstone of your universe, and you love to organize data into categories. You will work toward your perfect body if you are convinced that it will help you think, learn, and organize your life better and serve your spiritual mission as an administrator of data.

Endocrine Effects: The third chakra is affected by, and affects, the pancreas, a gland that lies across the stomach region. The pancreas is responsible for producing insulin, a hormone necessary for digesting foods, especially sugars, as well as several other hormones that aid growth and digestion. If working improperly, the pancreas will cause numerous health issues, including digestive disturbances, diabetes, hyper- or hypoglycemia or other blood sugar challenges, and even heart disease. If one or more of these problems already affect you, don't be discouraged. Perfecting your body will encourage better health. If you are not in poor health, celebrate! Then follow the regime that will keep you healthy.

The pancreas manages energies other than physical; it also processes information about pleasure. Pancreas-based people must play. Unfortunately, many Thinkers prize thoughts over fun. An imbalance between pleasure and work creates disharmonious relationships between people, and also within the body. A problem in the pancreas (or any other digestive organ) causes discordance elsewhere. A Thinker might remember that the perfect body takes more than counting calories or judiciously exercising; it requires a joyful pursuit of fun.

Diet: Eat for your pancreas's health, and you will have optimum health. Remember, however, that the pancreas is intimately connected to all your other digestive organs. If you overload the liver with toxic elements, such as alcohol, hydrogenated fats, or carcinogens, your pancreas (and all your other organs) will be adversely affected, and you will soon be bloated, fat, and depressed.

Thinker foods come in all varieties and colors, but many of the foods best suited for Thinkers are yellow. They thrive on foods derived from corn, squash, beans, poultry, papaya, pineapple, and other fruits that provide enzymes for good digestion. Just as important are factors like diet regulation and the reasons for eating.

Thinkers must eat with regularity, and they often flourish by grazing, or eating several small meals a day. The mammoth meals of the Manifester or the uncontrolled cravings of the Feeler are not for you. If you overload your system with fats, proteins, or starches you will suffer the consequences. In addition, Thinkers prosper when they consider their reasons for eating. Food holds energy. Popcorn eaten when you are angry will create more anger within your system, and probably stomach or gallbladder trouble as well. Donuts digested as a remedy for love troubles might create ulcers, as well as a potbelly!

Exercise: Motivate a Thinker to exercise, and you have signed up a gym member for life! Thinkers thrive on schedules, and they respond magnificently to routine exercise. This means that your perfect body is best achieved with an organized and thorough exercise plan, to include aerobic activity three days a week and weight-lifting, stretching, Pilates, yoga, or some other anaerobic activity the other two days a week. Circuit training is ideal for the dedicated Thinker, who likes to follow the same ritual every day or week. To support the pleasure-seeking needs of Thinkers, I also recommend dancing, whether it is ballroom, tap dance, or aerobic exercise.

Pitfalls and False Pleasures:
  • Meticulous perfectionism. A too-precise Thinker might starve, overexercise, or criticize him- or herself into a psychologically or physically life-threatening state.

- Excuses. You are so good at thinking that you could easily think of a thousand good reasons for putting off your health program.
- Mental madness. Analysis is good; being a perfectionist is not.
- Inflexibility. It is great to brush your hair a hundred times before going to bed, but will you lay sleepless when camping if you lack a comb? Perfectionism does not make a perfect body.
- Digestive issues. The third chakra influences most of the body's digestive organs, including the spleen, pancreas, stomach, liver, gallbladder, and parts of the esophagus, and it affects the intestines, kidneys, adrenals, and the heart. Poor eating habits, stress, self-esteem problems, fear, and bad attitudes can lead to the diseases mentioned earlier, such as hypo- or hyperglycemia and diabetes, heart arrhythmia, ulcers, immune disorders, chronic fatigue, fibromyalgia, and other problems with any digestive glands.
- Substance addictions. Thinkers who hate their jobs are highly susceptible to addictions or allergies to stimulants, including coffee, carbonated beverages, and products with NutraSweet. Caffeine keeps you going when your body says slow down. Carbonation makes you feel happy when you are not. In addition, NutraSweet provides a false sense of sweetness in an otherwise sour situation. Other third chakra temptations include corn- or grain-processed alcohols such as certain types of vodka, beer, and wine coolers. These types of addictions cover up buried anxieties and self-esteem issues.
- Action addictions. Thinkers can be susceptible to workaholism; obsessive-compulsive behaviors such as hand washing, excessive organization, anorexia, bulimia, and binge-purge cycles; and excessively judgmental attitudes, all behaviors that cloak a fear of being unacceptable or powerless in a scary world.
- Sensitivities. Food sensitivities are frequent, as an overstrained pancreas eventually becomes unable to break down simple sugars or even complex carbohydrates, leading to allergies or sensitivities to corn, citric acid, MSG or other preservatives, sugar, honey, NutraSweet, breads, grains, fruit, fats, and even minerals.

• Self-esteem issues. Traumas experienced from ages two and a half to four and a half can be the root. Frequently, these confidence-reducing experiences involve boundary violations, in which authority figures were too rigid or too lax with limitations. Either way, we can fail to develop self-trust. Lack of self-empowerment can lead to lack of success in work and relationships.

Success Tips:

• Diet. The Thinker should consider eating several small meals a day and limiting the use of simple sugars, fruits, NutraSweet, caffeine, and sweetened carbonated beverages. For a solid start in weight loss, consider a program called Diet Directives, which limits portions (see page 137). Eat eighty-five bites of food a day, even if these bites include a bit of apple pie or creamed corn. Structured programs and processes are perfect for the contract-minded Thinker.

• Supplements. Because of their pancreatic dependency, Thinkers can benefit especially from supplemental enzymes. Depending upon your health issues, you might select a sugar/starch enzyme (for the stomach and pancreas) or a fat enzyme (for the liver and gallbladder). Liquid minerals, especially those ionized with sea salt, can be beneficial. Add other supplements as needed; for instance, milk thistle, as well as a mixture of cayenne pepper, olive oil, lemon juice, parsley, ginger, and pectin, can cleanse the liver. If you are bothered by anxiety due to an overstressed mind (which can sometimes be misdiagnosed as attention deficit disorder), work with a natural care physician and explore whether you need increased inositol, magnesium, choline, and lecithin. (Note: Inositol increases the effectiveness of vitamin B and is often used to calm people with ADD.)

• Liver watch. The emotional causes of alcoholism often stem from first-chakra issues, but the physical condition originates in the liver. Certain individuals and ethnic groups lack a liver enzyme necessary to break down alcohol. Studies have shown that individuals missing this enzyme are allergic to alcohol and are prone to alcoholism. If alcoholism is a weakness in your family, consider yourself lacking in this enzyme and therefore unable to tolerate alcohol. Also, consider limiting your use of chemicals and drugs that damage the liver, including Tylenol.

- Change the type of oils you consume. Healthy fats are the key to healthy organs. Eliminate hydrogenated fats and consider using the following oils in supplement form or, if appropriate, as cooking oil: olive, macadamia nut, grapeseed, black currant, cranberry, evening primrose, avocado, sesame, coconut, fish, and flaxseed.

- Eating disorders. Boys and men are now joining the crush of women and girls endangered by eating disorders, which include anorexia, bulimia, and binge-purge. Psychologically, many of these issues are linked to control issues initiated in the third chakra between ages two and a half and four and a half, and developed throughout a lifetime of the culture's tendency toward perfectionism. If your standards are too high, then so is your level of personal shame, two factors that can result in the type of perfectionism that leads to food addictions and problems. Work with a specialized professional if you are concerned about an eating disorder, and be sure to work also with a holistic nutritionist or naturopath to test for food allergies and sensitivities, which almost always accompany eating disorders.

- Accept ambiguity. Thinkers like thoughts, especially those that line up in orderly columns. Life is messier than a balance sheet, however. Ultimately, the only cure for one's fears is the acceptance of ambiguity. Start by considering that there might really be a higher power that can handle what you cannot.

- Forgive. Can you forgive others for not being as perfect as you want them to be? Can you forgive yourself for setting standards that are impossible to achieve?

- Forget the "perfect" perfect body. Your ideal body will not be exactly perfect, just perfect for you.

- Auric close-down. Thinkers can be overwhelmed by life's details, as well as the infinite number of ideas, thoughts, and concepts afloat in the universe. Close your aura to energies that don't contribute to your purpose and well-being by envisioning it as a yellow net with white lights at the corners. Ask the Divine to program the white lights to deflect information that does not pertain to you.

- Use your intuition. Enormously logical, Thinkers also possess the capacity for intuitive knowing. This inner sensing, or mental empathy, interprets psychic information. Turn your perfect body program over to your intuition, and let it guide you.

Style: Thinkers are extraordinarily practical in dress and style. You are not going to find a Thinker changing a flat tire while wearing a ball gown or tuxedo. He or she would change into overalls first. Your look is planned and precise.

Supportive Assistants:
- Divine guidance. Ask the Divine to appoint for you a guide that will inform you empathetically about your perfect body program. To access energies to help you develop and live within your perfect body, ask the Divine to program your third auric field with positive beliefs. These beliefs will attract spiritual and real-life energies to encourage your perfect body.
- Grounding yourself. Weight issues often result from energetically operating from the solar plexus rather than the tenth chakra, which is underneath your feet. If you concentrate your consciousness in your stomach, you will become exhausted easily, strain your digestive organs, and crave carbohydrates, caffeine, and sweetened carbonated beverages as stimulants. To break yourself of poor energetic habits, place your sense of self in your feet and picture the energies of love and sustenance rising upward through your entire body. Do this four times daily for the best results.

Chakra Four: Relater
Spiritual Motivation: Relaters understand the interrelationship between all things, and they are most apt to develop their perfect bodies if they understand that physical health assures a long life full of love.

Endocrine Effects: Until recently, Western medicine failed to perceive what Eastern practices and ancient mystical healers have long known: The heart is a major endocrine gland. In fact, many researchers are beginning to believe that the heart is *the* major endocrine gland, its rhythm and protocol determining the well-being of all the other hormone-producing organs, including the brain. Certainly, we know that the heart produces 50,000 times more femtoteslas—a measure of the electromagnetic field—than does the brain, so the heart cannot be overlooked as the electrical center of the body.

Nourish the heart and you nourish the fourth-chakra person. According to research by organizations including the Institute of HeartMath in California, the heart not only requires tangibles like nutrients and exercise, but it is also affected by intangibles such as love, faith, and hope.

In addition to the heart, the fourth chakra also rules the lungs and the breasts. If your heart is happy, your fourth chakra will radiate healing energies throughout your entire body.

Diet: Think "heart healthy" and you have the perfect Relater diet. Heart-based diets also sustain all other bodily organs. In general, a heart-healthy diet is closest to the Mediterranean diet that has become popular in recent years, a diet based on fatty fish, lean poultry, reduced amounts of red meat, olive oil, vegetables, and whole grains. I have summarized a few heart-healthy tips from Dr. David Williams, whose products and newsletters can be obtained over the Internet at www.drdavidwilliams.com, and added my own.

- Eggs. The choline and lecithin in eggs moves cholesterol through the bloodstream and also calms brain activity. Some stores now sell lecithin-enriched eggs for an added boost.
- Onions. These keep blood pressure and cholesterol counts normal.
- Soybeans. Soybeans support a healthy heart and can mitigate some of the effects of menopause. One type of fermented soybean contains an enzyme called nattokinase. When tested with other foods for their ability to promote healthy circulation, nattokinase comes in first.

- Nuts. Three ounces of nuts a day are great for your heart. Nuts are full of minerals like selenium and essential fatty acids like omega-3 and omega-9 fatty acids.
- More omega fats. Although the average diet provides more omega-6 than omerga-3, you need a 4:1 ratio of omega-6 to omega-3 fatty acids. Two excellent sources of omega-3 fats are flax, best obtained through cold-pressed flaxseed oil, and fish, especially fatty fishes like salmon, sardines, and tuna.
- Avoid processed foods. They contain "metabolic disrupters"—food additives like nitrates, MSG, preservatives, white flour, and white sugar, which disturb healthy functions throughout the body.
- For heart health, think green—and pink and gold. The heart chakra begins as green in childhood and evolves to pink and then to gold with maturity. These colors all indicate heart-healthy foods. Greens such as broccoli that are good for the heart help ward off cancer as well. Pink foods include salmon, and gold adds various heart-happy spices and herbs, including cayenne pepper, garlic, hawthorn, and turmeric. Support for the lungs includes peppermint, oregano, and shiitake mushrooms (to reduce common lung ailments, such as mold, bacterial, or yeast problems). Quercetin and other antioxidants are good for breast support.

Exercise: Spend time to make your heart beat faster and you will enjoy a longer life! You have to increase your heart rate for at least thirty minutes at a time, three times a week, to dilate and expand your blood vessels so they remain elastic. Just about any exercise will help, including fast walking, swimming, jogging, bicycling, dancing—and even prolonged sex!

Pitfalls and False Pleasures:
- Central health issues. The chest area is prey to several major, life-threatening ailments, including heart disease, the number two cause of natural death among Americans after cancer. Lung cancer is the leading cancer killer, and breast cancer will strike one of every eight women in America. Other fourth-chakra illnesses include asthma, bronchitis, leukemia, and emphysema.

- Caretaking. To caretake means to take care of others' needs to your own detriment. Caretaking is not only a psychological issue, but an energetic one as well. Everything is made of energy, including others' issues and feelings. Relaters frequently absorb others' negativities, issues, and problems, thinking that this will heal their loved ones' problems. You cannot heal an issue that is not yours to heal; you will simply make yourself ill.
- Love addictions. If a relationship makes you feel bad, especially about yourself, it is not love. It is an addiction.
- Physical addictions. Sugar is the number one addiction in the United States; most people consume about ten tablespoons a day. Relaters crave sugar for a different reason than do Feelers. Feelers' issues are related to their feelings, while Relaters' issues center on a perceived lack of love. Other addictions include wine, which alleviates loneliness; chocolate, which mirrors romantic feelings; cigarettes, which serve as false companions and cover grief; and inhalant drugs, which substitute for the Great Spirit.
- Giving-receiving imbalance. To cope with childhood lack, especially perceptions locked in from the ages of four and a half to six and a half, many Relaters develop an imbalanced giver-receiver pattern. Givers lose themselves in relationships to avoid their own needs and pain. Receivers take from others in the hope that they will not be abandoned.

Success Tips:
- Quit smoking. Smoking is the number one controllable contributor to heart disease and cancer. Almost 90 percent of all lung cancers can be traced to smoking. Besides endangering your life, smoking ruins your skin, yellows your teeth, and causes malnutrition. Do you need assistance to quit smoking? Try hypnotherapy to uncover to your underlying grief issues; join a support group; and work with a medical professional to obtain needed antidepressants or other therapies.
- Quit sugar. Sugar is a poor substitute for love. Try love instead. If you have a sweet tooth, consider replacements like plant-based

Stevia (see page 137), or molasses, which contains antioxidants and minerals, or a piece of dark, cocoa-based chocolate.

- Drink water. You need at least eight to ten glasses of water a day to cleanse your system.
- Eat for your heart. Reread the "Diet" section above; eating a healthy diet is a form of self-love.
- Drink tea. Green teas are great for the lungs, black teas are especially healing for the heart, white teas open spiritual energies, and red tea is a terrific antioxidant.
- Consume healthy fats. Eat enough omega-3 fatty acids; eating salmon three to four times a week (choose wild) actually alleviates arrhythmia and reduces arterial inflammation. Supplement with omega fats and alpha lipoic acids, and consider cooking in olive oil or grapeseed oil.
- Supplement. Besides the spices, herbs, and supplements listed under "Diet," I also recommend checking out CoQ10, folic acid, selenium, red grape juice, and, if you drink alcohol, controlled amounts of red wine, preferably organic and without preservatives. Cleansing the liver is beneficial if you are susceptible to heart disease; consider B vitamins, inositol, choline, and lecithin, N-acetyl cysteine (NAC), omega-3 fatty acids and omega-6 fatty acids, and milk thistle. Consider magnesium supplements and a liquid supplement program. Remember to consult with your doctor about any supplement program.
- Detoxify emotions. Emotions often clutter the heart. Analyze and express your feelings daily and again at night; limit your exposure to toxic people, newspapers, news shows, or relationships; and promote self-care.
- Stop caretaking. I recommend reading *Codependent No More* by Melody Beattie (Hazelden), which does an excellent job of explaining the stress that codependent relationships cause. If you are prone to bad relationships, join a support group, like Al-Anon for codependents to alcoholics, or CoSA for codependents to sexual addicts.
- Do you have asthma or breathing problems? Consider seeing a chiropractor, and get evaluated for dorsal vertebrae malfunctions,

almost always present with asthma and certain other problems. Test also for fungus in the lungs or candida in the body.

- Reconsider the assumption that you are broken. The heart cannot be broken, for it is always cleansed and renewed by the fountain of divine love that flows through it.

- Worship. The "attitude of gratitude" is the best all-around prescription for healing heart pain, physical or emotional. Give thanks, and you will receive more for which to be thankful.

- Pray, meditate, and contemplate. To pray is to communicate to the Divine. To meditate is to allow responses to come. To contemplate is to acknowledge the presence of divine grace. Ask the Divine to help you formulate your perfect body. Listen and await the responses, and then receive the unconditional love that you need in order to follow your perfect body program.

- Breathe. Your circulatory and respiratory systems depend upon oxygen, as do all intracellular processes. To perform healing breath work, breathe in for four counts and hold for four, then release for five counts. Do this for two minutes at a time.

- For women. Follow the tips listed under the sections "Diet" and "Exercise" and consider these ideas. Use the best of allopathic medicine. Schedule annual Pap smears, mammograms, and necessary heart checks. If you are going to be a new mother, breastfeed if possible. Breastfeeding for more than six months significantly reduces your chances of getting breast cancer. Review the advice already given about broccoli, and add Brussels sprouts to your list of frequently eaten vegetables; both contain sulforaphane, a compound the hinders the growth of breast cancer cells in the lab. Take extra mineral supplements, because under stress, women burn vast amounts of minerals. If you take B vitamins, consider taking a zinc tablet at the same time. If you have heart problems, check with your health practitioner about taking extra magnesium, as magnesium is one of the major deficiencies found in women with heart disease. Take enough calcium as well. Learn that loving yourself comes first; many women are trained to help others before themselves.

- For men. Maybe you are one of the few men who was taught how to feel his feelings when growing up, but chances are that it is still a challenge for you to actually share them. Feelings that are never shared become, eventually, a time bomb. Heart disease is linked to repressed feelings, as well as to other tangible factors. Try aromatherapy to put your mind at ease and open your heart. The scents of vanilla, cinnamon, and baking bread are known to be relaxing to men.

- Practice auric expansion. Having an open fourth auric field is equivalent to reaching into the universe for love with an open hand. Imagine pink or gold light emanating 360 degrees from the center of your heart. The core of this blazing sun is white. This white energy is divine grace, which sustains your own spiritual heart. As the light extends, notice that it transforms anything that is unloving or harmful to you into sparks that disappear into the vast unknown. Imagine that this expanding energy transmutes all internal toxins, negative feelings, and wastes, even as it alters the environment around you.

- Invite grace. After practicing the auric extension, welcome the gifts of love. With divine grace, your perfect body can unfold like a plant would. As you welcome in the warmth, allow the Divine to bestow the blessings of the universe, for surely you are a blessing unto the world as well.

Style: The Relater dresses to fit in. You do not conform because you are shallow or boring; instead, you value comfort and good manners. You will call ahead and ask about the mode of attire out of respect for a party host. Then you will select attire that lets you play on the floor with the children or the kittens hidden in the kitchen! Consider also clothes that are fluid, colorful, comfortable, and classy.

Supportive Assistants:
- Collaboration. You like to relate, so ask your partner or a friend to follow the same regimen as you.
- Grief therapy. The heart is often our receptacle of grief and sorrow. The most important way to keep your chest happy is to release

grievances, grief, and sorrow, including ancient pains, old emotions, and false beliefs. Work toward forgiving.

• The Divine. The Divine is the major guardian of your heart. Learn how to surrender the self-appointed job of being the world's healer, and let God be God.

• Others' love. Yes, other people have hurt you. You have probably caused a few heartbreaks yourself. You have reason to block your heart to giving or receiving love, but consider that an energetically blocked heart leads to a physically blocked heart. The Divine is your vertical connection to unconditional love. People (and all living beings) compose your horizontal connection to unconditional love. People might love imperfectly, but their divine spirits love with perfection. Accept that the human delivery of love might be imperfect, but love is still love.

Chakra Five: Communicator

Spiritual Motivation: As a Communicator, you are a vessel of truth. You usher heaven onto earth, whether it is through speaking, teaching, learning, talking, writing, singing, preaching, or composing. Your body is a conduit of the higher truths you seek to share with others. Develop it as a means to communicate for the Great Spirit.

Endocrine Effects: A Communicator's chief endocrine gland is the thyroid, a small organ in the throat area. The thyroid secretes hormones that control metabolism and growth.

There are many facets of communicating. Consider the esoteric functions of the fifth chakra and, therefore, the thyroid gland. The fifth chakra is the point for channeling higher truths. Messages from the beyond enter through the back side of the throat chakra, and are then focused into audible expressions through the front side. All major world religions were formulated through this process, as well as the world's library of literature, musical compositions, philosophies, and teachings. If you keep your thyroid healthy and strong, you assist the process of psychic and sensory communication.

There are health hazards to this fifth chakra's channeling function. Psychic elements can strain the body. To work, the thyroid taps into deeper adrenal and first-chakra fire energies, which can injure the throat area if overused. Fanatical Communicators, those overly devoted to their causes, are the most affected by this challenge. Overstimulation of the fire element can potentially lead to hyperthyroidism, an overproduction of thyroid hormones that causes hyperactivity, weight loss, sweating palms, exhaustion, fast heartbeat, insomnia, and a racing mind. Conversely, lack of fire or passion results in loss of hope and hypothyroidism, an underproduction of thyroid hormones characterized by weight gain, exhaustion, depression, cold hands or feet, food allergies, and insomnia. Hypothyroidism can also occur if you are hyperthyroid for so long that your thyroid burns out.

Some Communicators are prone to negative interference or overstimulation by invisible beings (like being possessed or haunted), and they can be by hyper- and hypothyroid at the same time. The body, overrun by alien forces, gives up and becomes exhausted. Some of the thyroid medical lab panels would therefore test as hypothyroid, and the adrenals will be low functioning. The soul continues to battle against invasion, efforts that can measure as hyperthyroidism on certain thyroid medical lab panels; the adrenals will also be overfunctioning. To maintain the correct weight, muscle tone, and a healthy frame of mind, a Communicator must always assess his or her thyroid health and use supplements, dietary controls, intuitive boundaries, or medication, if necessary, to maintain balance.

Diet: The ideal Communicator's cuisine is both nourishing and clearing. To prove my point, consider the numerous Communicators who have defied this advice in devotion to their craft. An example is author Ernest Hemingway, who survived on—and died because of—booze and cigarettes. Most Communicators must release the spell of their muse long enough to eat foods that nurture the body while alleviating stress.

Fifth-chakra foods are blue or deep red in color or are soothing to the throat. Blueberries, blackberries, cherries, red cabbage, and beets flush toxins and encourage a functional lymph system. High in vitamin C and minerals, they provide fuel for the Communicator's intense fire and fiber to cleanse the system. Softer foods like soup, mashed potatoes, and steamed vegetables provide nutrients and calm the fire stoking the Communicator's métier.

Exercise: Given the sometimes-anxious nature of the dedicated Communicator, one of the best exercises for a Communicator is walking. Walking evens out inconsistent energies in the body and assuages the soul, as does dancing. Exercise involving tempo and rhythm capture the attention of the auditory Communicator also.

Pitfalls and False Pleasures:
- Physical maladies. Communicators can experience problems with the thyroid, as well as the larynx, throat, ears, jaw, teeth, and the back of the neck, and they exhibit tendencies toward anemia, blood deficiencies, lymph restrictions, goiter, and adrenal exhaustion.
- Congestion. Dairy and sugars can clog the Communicator's thoughts and throat, as well as lead to sugar highs and lows.
- Addictions and compulsions. Communicators are orally fixated, which can lead to smoking, mindless eating or drinking, and gum (or even pencil) chewing. They can also be addicted to work, seeking an ever-higher thrill or connection to their muse.
- Nervousness or lethargy. Depending upon the state of the thyroid, a Communicator can become easily overwrought or sluggish.
- Psychic susceptibility. There are millions of auditory psychic sources. The Communicator can become prey to any of these, for good or for ill.

Success Tips:
- Nutritional supportive actions. Eat foods with plenty of antioxidants and minerals, and consider supplementing your diet with antioxidants as well. Try a liquid mineral or vitamin supplement; up to 50 percent of certain nutrients carried in liquids dissolve in the mouth. Take iron tablets or eat red meats if you are anemic. Avoid milk or dairy products if they create mucus.
- Drink water. Nothing beats a Communicator's oral compulsion like keeping something healthy in his or her mouth. Try water

and tea—or even sugarless gum—instead of sweetened carbonated beverages and cigarettes.

- Eliminate sugar. Sugar corrodes thyroid tissue and plays havoc with blood sugar, creating mood swings. Try sucking on sugar-free candies, drinking cider with cinnamon, or using Stevia, (see page 137) a natural sweetener, instead of white sugar.
- Listen and learn. Consider listening to music or books on tape. Learning soothes your nerves while motivating healthy behavior.
- Kiss. Your highly sensitive mouth is one of your most erotic zones. Kissing will raise your endorphins, and therefore your metabolism and your happiness level.
- Say no. And yes. One of the major challenges for Communicators is to be honest with their "yesses" and their "nos." Say what you mean.
- Turn off the voices. If you are overwhelmed by the interference or intrusion of negative invisible beings, look for intuitive or spiritual training to stop the overload.
- Talk it through. Problems of any nature might arise from issues incurred during ages six and a half to eight and a half, when the throat chakra opened, or from experiences causing you to shut off your voice. Find a professional therapist.

Style: Many Communicators ignore the basics of contemporary fashion, and sometimes fashion in general. When involved in their craft, they do not care what they look like. A Communicator's style emerges when presenting their art form to the world, at which point they conform to professional standards (or lack thereof). An orchestral conductor will appear in a tux when on stage; a poet will play the part of the nonconformist artist and wear a haphazard outfit when reciting.

Supportive Assistants:
- A gatekeeper. Ask the Divine to appoint you a gatekeeper, a spiritual being that will screen positive from negative entities and energies and inform you of the steps necessary for unlocking your perfect body.
- Celestial beings. Entities and angels that serve the Divine are always available to heal your wounds and encourage your growth

and achievements. Ask the Divine to assign you the guidance that will work for you.

- Great Communicators of the past. History is replete with great Communicators, whose works are still alive. Nothing supports a Communicator more than the thoughts, music, or knowledge of their predecessors, from Mozart to Plato to Tolstoy. Study these people, and ask the Divine to send you their advice intuitively.

Chakra Six: Visionary

Spiritual Motivation: Magicians pull rabbits out of hats; Visionaries form reality out of air. Feelers might paint with brushes and oils, but Visionaries do so with color and ideas. To achieve their perfect body, Visionaries must believe in it; they can then manifest reality out of wishes, hopes, and stars. If you're a Visionary, know that if you can dream it, you can materialize it.

Endocrine Effects: The pituitary gland rests in the base of the brain, manufacturing hormones supporting bone growth, sexual maturation, and metabolism. Some scientists consider the pituitary the master gland; at the least, it is formative in regulating almost all sexual hormone activities. The pituitary affects Visionaries' bodies in many ways.

If physically healthy, the pituitary gland will enable an active mind, strategic thinking, solid self-esteem, a positive body image, inner vision, and a lean, healthy body. If the pituitary gland is unhealthy, it can cause sluggish thinking, meandering thoughts, self-loathing, a negative body image, lack of vision, and potential weight problems and hormone irregularities. A Visionary is always challenged by a vulnerability to stress and poor physical endurance. They are able to compensate using their astonishing ability to set and achieve goals. Serious distortions in self-image caused by negative beliefs can also cause warped inner vision and the psychic susceptibility to entities creating hallucinations or fantastical mirages.

Diet: Pituitary health necessitates the same foods required by the Feeler and the Relater, with an emphasis on fish, seafood, or vegetable proteins. Purple foods will strengthen your immune system. Consider black or red grapes or berries and juices, and other vitamin and mineral-rich natural fruits and vegetables. The pituitary gland is especially affected by hallucinogens and visual stimulants, including medicinal plants used in other cultures for visioning, and cocoa.

Exercise: The most beneficial exercise program for the Visionary is one that moves and builds all parts of the body weekly. Design a training program that will increase muscle while sculpting attractive curves and edges. You could combine weight lifting and walking, or perhaps rowing and running. You are going for an overall attractive look.

Pitfalls and False Pleasures:
- Physical challenges. The foremost complaint of the pituitary-driven Visionary is sexual hormone imbalances. Pituitary problems can throw off the ovaries, testes, adrenals, and thyroid, among other glands. Other issues can include problems with emotional and mental health, metabolic disturbances, and problems with the eyes, including vision.
- Addictions and desires. It is possible to become obsessed with having a "perfect" perfect body. Visually oriented, Visionaries are liable to a neurotic obsession with appearance, weight, and looks. Lack of self-acceptance can lead to body dysmorphia, a distorted body image, and potentially to anorexia, bulimia, or addictions to specific foods. Visionaries with high stress and anger can also become shopaholics.
- Chocolate. Chocolate is not bad; it has anticarcinogenic properties and can soothe the most frantic of hormones. However, not all chocolates are equal in quality. Most chocolate contains unnecessary additives, caffeine, dairy products, and white sugar. These ingredients can cause blood sugar problems and therefore mood swings and cravings—and too much of anything puts on weight.

- Missed opportunities. Driven by goals, Visionaries can forget to smell, pick, and sometimes plant flowers along the way. Happiness lies in the here and now, not just the future. If you live only for the future, you will never enjoy the present.
- Unwanted visions. Visionaries instinctively gaze through the veils between the worlds, seeing what others cannot see. This psychic sense is called visual sympathy or clairvoyance, which means "clear seeing," and it accounts for insight, revelation, inner vision, and the receiving of visual messages and future predictions. If uncontrolled, this psychic ability can overwhelm the Visionary with unwanted, frightening, or even dangerous visions.

Success Tips:
- Eat greens. The minerals in leafy green vegetables will help keep you balanced and focused.
- Visualize red. When your eyes perceive red or orange colors, your pituitary gland boosts energy production. Buy those rose-colored glasses if you need more energy for life and exercise!
- See the sun. Studies show that people consume up to 1,500 more calories per day in the winter. Why? It seems that up to 20 percent of Americans suffer from seasonal affective disorder, or SAD, which causes mild to severe depression from a reduction in dopamine and serotonin. The pituitary is greatly affected by the presence or absence of these hormones. Visionaries should get some direct sunshine every day for at least ten minutes between 10 A.M. and 2 P.M.
- Adjust the lighting. Research has determined that overweight people eat more food in brightly lit settings. Visionaries are so visual that they might want to dim the lights when eating.
- Hide your food. According to various studies, foods on lower cabinet shelves are consumed more often than those on higher shelves. Conceal those tempting desserts and calorie-laden treats, and opt for carrots and celery instead.
- Follow your nose. Your senses of sight and smell are intertwined. Discourage cheating on your diet by avoiding bakeries or other locations with seductive sights. Entice your palate with healthy

foods that smell great. Light candles that smell like cinnamon, ginger, or oranges to make you feel full and satiated.

• Turn off the television. People eat more when sitting in front of the television.

• Try color. A Visionary's mood alters with color hues. If you are wearing red, you will feel bold and desirous; blue will bring out the student in you. Try using these colors in clothing, decorating, table dressing, or exercise attire to call forth your perfect body:

Red	Attunes your sexuality and hormones and motivates you to exercise.
Orange	Assuages feelings, staving off emotional eating.
Yellow	Keeps you thinking positively and on track with a diet and exercise program. Visualize yellow if you want to identify a belief that will unfold your perfect body.
Green	Heals heart wounds, which can dampen the Visionary's enthusiasm for looking his or her best.
Blue	Attracts spiritual guidance to assist you on your quest.
Purple	Imagine this color and then ask which steps to take next on your venture into your own perfection.
White	Wash your body daily with an imaginary flow of white light, to cleanse you of confusion and hormone imbalances and to alleviate mental strain.
Black	This color will help you hide; use black if you are feeling exposed to help you stay calm.
Gold	The "miracle color"; imagine or wear this color for divine help with your perfect body venture.

• Decorate for success. Visionaries respond to the textures, sights, colors, and fashion in their environment. Water fountains soothe overtaxed nerves. A subdued décor decreases food cravings. Make sure that your bedroom is an abode of peace; Visionaries' sleep cycles are greatly affected by their surroundings.

• Think proportion—in everything. Eat balanced meals. If you wear one color on the top part of your body, wear the same color on the lower part of your body.

- Exercise each muscle group. Exercise the same amount each day. Your calling card to success is proportion and harmony.
- Use your connection to the Divine. First thing in the morning, before starting your day, connect with the Divine. Imagine your perfect body. Now ask the Divine to reveal a picture describing today's step for manifesting that goal. A Visionary's success follows his or her mind's eye. In fact, just two minutes of positive visioning can erase up to 65 percent of anxiety-triggered worry, according to British studies.[3]
- Find an inspirational picture. Use your physical eyes, and not just your inner one, to achieve your perfect body. Find a photograph that embodies the perfection you are seeking. Place this picture where you will constantly see it.
- Use a traffic light for making decisions. Imagine a traffic light and then pose yourself a simple question. Ask about that rich chocolate dessert. Green means "yes," red is "no," and yellow says, "ask a new question," or "think of something better." What color lights up in your mind's eye? Follow the advice given, or ask a new question for more clarity.
- Screen the visions. Some Visionaries are overwhelmed by predictions of future disaster. Ask the Divine to establish a filter system in your sixth auric field, and to assign a gatekeeper or a guiding angel to screen out harmful revelations.

Style: You have a style of your own, which is certainly dramatic, and probably also classy. You prefer a classic and elegant look. You will offset red leather pants with a white tuxedo shirt, for example, not a green polka-dotted top. Settle on a signature look, including mainstay colors and accessories.

Supportive Assistants:
- An interior decorator. You are the visual protégé of the chakra system. Hire someone to design an environment for who you are becoming, not for who you currently are. Also consider using a feng shui expert. A specialist in the art of energy and placement, this master can create an environment that will support your perfect body goals.

- A shopping advisor. You behave best when you look your best. Find someone to assess your needs and style and to keep you on target with clothing purchases that support your greater goals.
- A coach. Visionaries love to plan, but sometimes it is nice to have a partner who can reduce long-range plans into daily tasks. Either hire a professional or ask a friend to help you. Talk daily about goals, achievements, failures, and needs.
- A spiritual guide. Your visual sense is an incredible asset. Use it. Ask the Divine to appoint you a guide or gatekeeper to inform you through revelation, insight, visions, or dreams of what you need to know to unfold your perfect body.

Chakra Seven: Spiritualist

Spiritual Motivation: There is one spiritual absolute for the Spiritualist: to serve God. An underdeveloped Spiritualist will typically indulge in negative first-chakra behaviors, such as sex, alcohol, work, or other addictions. Disavowing all things physical, an overzealous Spiritualist might ignore the body in a militant attempt to be "good." To have a perfect body, the Spiritualist must acknowledge the presence of the Divine in the physical world and take care of his or her physical body.

Endocrine Effects: The pineal gland is one of the most magical and mysterious organs of the human body. Scientists know that it produces melatonin, serotonin, and other hormones necessary for the regulation of mood and sleep. It also manufactures DMT, a chemical connected to spiritual experiences. Some researchers believe that the pineal is the master gland of the body, and if it is fully functioning, it opens our higher-learning brain centers to their true potential.

As a pineal-oriented person, a Spiritualist is prone to problems like sleep and mood disorders and hormonal imbalances. If open to the Divine and his or her own spiritual purpose, the Spiritualist's pineal gland is apt to be healthy, at which point it opens to several major spiritual gifts. These include:

- The gift of prophecy or knowledge of divine will.
- Spiritual awareness or perceptions of angels, ghosts, and other entities.
- Access to spiritual energies, such as those that promote healing or inspiration.

Your perfect body will absolutely require the full opening of the pineal gland in accordance with your highest spiritual values.

Diet: Think moderation and you will be healthy! Unfortunately, many Spiritualists tend toward one of two extremes: culinary asceticism or total overindulgence. A Spiritualist would do well to adopt the doctrine of moderation.

In general, a Spiritualist's perfect body requires foods that are white, chemically pure, grown in the sun, and mineral-rich. These include white fish, white asparagus, chicken, garbanzo beans, nuts, white beans, potatoes, turnips, pastas, and various sun-ripened fruits and vegetables, such as tomatoes, zucchini, cantaloupe, oranges, lemons, and pineapple. Olive oil is the ideal fat, and white wines and green or white teas are good accompaniments. The Mediterranean diet of seafood, olive oil, and vegetables, also appropriate for the Relater, is perfect for the Spiritualist.

Exercise: The ideal Spiritualist exercise takes place in the sun. You probably have seasonal affective disorder (SAD), which means that you will become depressed unless you enjoy at least ten minutes of full-spectrum light a day, preferably from direct sun. Spiritualists should also enjoy full-body exercise whenever possible, such as running, walking, swimming, skiing, or ball games. Spiritualists are famous for ignoring their body in favor of spiritual interests, but full-body movements encourage the unification of spirit and body.

Pitfalls and False Pleasures:
- Fanaticism. Immoderation causes tension and a weak body.
- Seclusion. *Pray* and *play* are almost the same words! Try play. It is a great cure for depression and boredom.

- A judgmental attitude. Spiritualism is only one of the eleven main chakra types. The world is full of people who praise the Divine and live spiritually by playing tennis or enjoying dinner with a friend. Judgments of others' ways of expression creates worry, which turns into anxiety and physical tension.

- Depression and anxiety. An unhealthy Spiritualist is highly susceptible to depression and anxiety. Some Spiritualists become depressed because of sleep disorders, which can be caused by SAD, chemical imbalances in the brain, heavy-metal toxicity, or an overly judgmental attitude. In general, lack of trust in the Divine leads to anxiety disorders, and a refusal to allow joy or to heal from the past can lead to depression.

- Purposelessness. Ironically, the Spiritualist is the most apt to feel unfulfilled and think that life holds no meaning. The seventh chakra invites everyone to open to his or her purpose, especially between the ages of fourteen and twenty-one. However, Spiritualists are hard on themselves, seldom believing that they have lived up to the Divine's standards. The belief that they have fallen short leads to a lack of personal, professional, or relationship satisfaction.

- Relationship unhappiness. If purity becomes confused with perfection, Spiritualists can hold themselves and sometimes others to impossible ideologies. This creates relationship discord and pain.

- Physical problems. Seventh chakra issues can include certain learning disorders such as attention deficit disorder and auditory processing challenges; mental health issues including depression, anxiety, certain forms of schizophrenia, bipolar or manic depression, obsessive compulsive disorder, and multiple personality disorder; certain addictions such as alcoholism; brain tumors and other head challenges; and eating or exercising too much or too little. Pineal gland challenges can include depression and anxiety, heavy-metal toxicity, SAD, insomnia, and sun sensitivity.

Success Tips:
- Choose spirituality. Every major religion or spiritual discipline acknowledges the role of the body in housing the spirit. A poorly

treated body will not fulfill spiritual duties. Research and then recite the spiritual dogma that will encourage the emergence of your health and full beauty.

- Pray, meditate, and contemplate. Communication with the Divine through prayer, meditation, and contemplation is crucial to the Spiritualist's process. Ask the Divine to direct your body plan, and use these three methods daily to follow it.

- Get into the sunshine. If you cannot, use halogen lighting in an office, buy full-spectrum lights for your home, or sit under a sun lamp in the morning.

- Get inspired through exercise. Consider exercise as an extension of your prayer, meditation, or contemplation time. This will keep you motivated and counteract any sense that exercise is a waste of your time.

- Do a vision quest. Many ancient and indigenous cultures use the vision quest to help people open to their life purpose and connect with spiritual guidance. Obtain guidance from a native or spiritual leader or conduct your own quest by setting aside a short period of time, from one to three days, during which you sequester yourself, abstain from food or conduct a partial fast, and ask the Divine to reveal your purpose and spiritual guides to you. It is ideal to undergo such a quest alone and in nature, but you can even perform one in a hotel or at home! Prepare by praying the days and weeks before, and by performing an initial and closing sacred ceremony.

- See a specialist. If you are affected by any of the physical or mental health traumas of your chakra type, get help from professionals. Consider working with an expert in detoxification and especially heavy-metal chelation if you are depressed or anxious.

- Use supplements. Brain foods, medications, and supplements might be extraordinarily helpful to you, as long as you work with a professional for diagnosis and follow-up. Have your doctor consider amino acids such as taurine or GABA if you are over-stressed; herbs or supplements like SAM-e, 5HTP, or St. John's wort if you are depressed; phosphocholine, inositol, DHA, amino acids, or healthy fats and supplements if you are anxious or affected by conditions like attention deficit disorder; testing for food allergies and chemical sensitivities if you are affected by autism, attention deficit disorder, attention deficit hyperactivity disorder, or Asperger's syndrome; attending a sleep disorder clinic or using hypnotherapy, EMDR, emotional freedom treatment (EFT), or herbs like valerian and passion flower if you are affected by sleep disorders; and obtaining a neuro-medication like antidepressants or antianxiety drugs under the guidance of a psychiatrist if you are chemically imbalanced.

- Eat salmon. Studies are showing that eating salmon, tuna, or another EPA-enriched fish two to three times a week can be as effective as taking antidepressants. To avoid heavy-metal accumulation, buy wild fish.
- Bless your food. Food and water take on energy. Consider the work of Dr. M. Emoto of Japan, whose books describe the structural changes that take place in water that has been blessed. Bless the bounty of your table and you will receive blessings in return.
- Go for grace. If struggling with body care, ask for grace. Grace is the combined energy of divine love and power. Grace releases traumas and invites holy healing. It occurs when four ingredients are simultaneously present: holding compassion for yourself and others, and forgiving yourself and others. At the juncture of these steps, the Divine takes over and encourages miracles.

Style: Most Spiritualists conform in style to their religious or spiritual persuasion. Spiritualists dress like their fellow worshipers. Attire is functional, a way to promote your godly mission, but it is also a way to conform to the Divine. A church pastor with a large teenage congregation might boast piercings, tattoos, and a Harley Davidson motorcycle, but most Spiritualists tend toward the conservative side of fashion. The key is to select a style that expresses your relationship with the Divine yet allows joy.

Supportive Assistants:

- A spiritual director. Spiritual directors might be pastors or priests, therapists or counselors, specially trained directors, or simply friends who provide spiritual insight. Spiritual directors go beyond everyday coaching and help you look at practical decisions in light of spiritual principles and values.

- A prayer chain. Spiritualists are mighty contributors to and benefactors from a prayer chain, a group of intercessory partners who ask the Divine to intercede for health and well-being. Join a prayer chain in your place of worship or start your own.

- Spiritual guides. Spiritualists are innately able to connect directly with the Divine as well as spiritual beings, including ghosts, guides, angels, and demons. Work with a trained spiritual director, intuitive teacher, or religious leader to learn how to use this ability correctly and safely, and then tap into it for body guidance.

Chakra Eight: Shaman

Spiritual Motivation: The Shaman is the maestro of mystery. Traversing the worlds of Nature, humankind, and magic, the Shaman blends energies of all worlds to create new ones. As a Shaman, this is your spiritual mission.

Think of the intense pressure involved in connecting so many universes, dimensions, and planes through your physical self. You *must* develop your perfect body, if only to bolster strength for this amazing endeavor! It is physically stressful to regulate so many energies simultaneously. The temptation is to borrow energies from other people to form your own perfect body.

As a Shaman, you can acquire powers from any resource, including others' energetic and physical bodies. "Stealing energy" leaves holes inside of others and provides you with a false sense of security. Issues of spiritual integrity must be faced in your personal development and perfect body plan. Mistakes in integrity boomerang, leaving the Shaman to bear the energetic damage. Eventually, all energetic wounds transform into physical ones.

Though you might not be spiritually responsible for all the dents incurred through the use of your gifts, you are vulnerable to energies not even noticed by other people, a threat that leads to only one solution: development of protection. Your perfect body must extend into the invisible realm, where you can attract energies useful to your endeavors but keep out harmful ones. Accomplishing this task requires special spiritual principles and practices, and often the use of ritual on a daily basis.

Endocrine Effects: All Shamans must safeguard and utilize their chief endocrine gland, the thymus. The thymus sits in the upper chest. Housed between the fourth and fifth chakras, it blends the healing powers of the heart center with the communication gifts of the throat chakra. Biologically, the thymus is one of the two main immune system organs, producing cells that defend the body against physical invaders. Here we see encapsulated the Shaman's challenge of being approachable yet defended. If your thymus is functioning appropriately, it will deflect physical marauders like viruses, bacteria, and allergens and energetic forces such as entities and curses, but it will attract powerful healing forces like universal energies and spiritual help.

Diet: Many Shamans love to make others think that they can eat anything, transmuting pizza into vitamins and chocolate into protein. Beware. The healthy Shaman—the one that wants full use of universal healing energies—indulges only in a healthy diet. The best diet is a heart-healthy diet with extra protein, as most Shamans run strong multidimensional energies through their heart and support their work with their adrenals.

The other dietary obstacle for many Shamans is the expected use of ceremonial substances. Around the world, Shamans coax healing, hallucinations, and help out of materials that others might consider dangerous. Here are a few of the substances used in ritual, and the mystical assumptions made about each:

- Sugar: Used for bonding and love, and to heal love wounds.
- Coffee: Stimulates and heals the nervous system.
- Tobacco: Opens the doors between worlds, and summons negative spirits that might be causing disease or disasters. Also used for protection against evil entities or energies.
- Chocolate: Kindles the magical "third eye" or sixth chakra for psychic vision, and heals false or destructive dreams and beliefs.

- Alcohol: Releases inhibitions and calls forth the negative entities, beliefs, or memories causing problems or illness.
- Hallucinogens: Inspires perceptions of the invisible and creates connections with helpful or harmful spirits.

Given that Shamans are as human as the other chakra types, it is little wonder that many Shamans suffer from illness, depression, and relationship troubles. Who can survive a diet of the above or the steady stream of harmful energies flowing unaltered through the body? Who can live with a Shaman who is always high—or low? The perceptive Shaman stops using the listed substances and instead works energetically, substituting healthy substances for the customary sacraments.

Following are suggestions of replacement substances for the unhealthy ones. These foods and substances compose the ideal shamanic diet.

Ritual Substances, Substitutes, or Counteractive Substances
- Sugar: Green vegetables, yams and sweet potatoes, pineapple, papaya, mangoes, coconut, lemon, apricots, parsley, apple cider vinegar, black or brown beans, and low-fat proteins, like fish or chicken; for healing the heart and protection from negative relationship energies, use teas and tinctures with pink yarrow; drink red tea for extra energy
- Coffee: Water, green tea with lemongrass or mint, or black tea applied topically (as in a bathtub) for entity release and protection
- Tobacco: Cayenne pepper, oregano, peppermint, spinach; for protection, use black tea topically or internally, and teas or tinctures of yellow yarrow
- Chocolate: Cocoa powder, organic maple syrup, molasses, dark organic chocolate, ginger, cinnamon, cloves, nutmeg, and flower essences, such as Bach flower remedies; for third eye protection, use teas or tinctures of white yarrow
- Alcohol: Red grape juice, dark berries, or cherries

- Hallucinogens: Aromatic spices, tinctures, and juices that are lightly fermented, apple juice with lemon and cinnamon; to inspire visions, use raw cocoa

In addition, the clever Shaman uses healthy fat products, like coconut, macadamia nut, cranberry, flaxseed, evening primrose, black currant, grapeseed, avocado, or olive oil.

Exercise: Shamans are challenged to develop two different sets of muscles, the long and the short. Long muscles lend elasticity and suppleness and allow for bending between the worlds. Short muscles provide bulk and strength and provide power against adversity. Therefore, Shamans are encouraged to undertake long-muscle exercises like stretching, yoga, Pilates, or tai chi three times a week, as well as short-muscle development, which includes weight lifting or heavy outdoor work, three times a week.

You can also divide your workouts between anaerobic and aerobic exercise. Anaerobic workouts (like weight lifting, calisthenics, and isometrics) tear muscle down, requiring the body to rebuild for Herculean might. Aerobic exercises (like running, walking, swimming, and dancing) promote cardiovascular health and endurance. Shamans are known for living in two worlds, and they must exercise for them both!

Pitfalls and False Pleasures:
- Sexual indulgence. Most Shamans have vast amounts of first-chakra energy, which is comprised of life energy and is often used sexually. Unfortunately, many Shamans employ sex to coax their partner's first-chakra red energy into their own veins. Unlimited sexual indulgence threatens close relationships, hurts others, and provides a false sense of power.
- Substance addictions. Too much of a bad thing is really bad.
- Ego. Many a Shaman has fallen prey to attacks of the ego that leave him or her feeling invulnerable and invincible. The types of tumbles experienced by egotistical Shamans can include illness

or death from addictions, entity interference or possession, and even illness or death from the curses of jealous competitors.

- Entity interference. This issue deserves particular mention. A Shaman weak in body (and soul) is apt to experience invasion from external entities, energies, and ghosts. Hosts of external energies often stimulate illness, heart problems, nervous system issues, hallucinations, paranoia, mood distortion, cravings, and even schizophrenia.

Success Tips:

- Quit. Good health requires abstinence from the unhealthy substances listed in the "Diet" section, with the exception of the rare piece of chocolate, which ought to be dark and organic.

- Cleanse. If you have struggled with cravings for less than healthy foods, try the shamanic diet as a way to cleanse. This diet eliminates all salt, red meat, sugar, caffeine, and dairy products in favor of yams or sweet potatoes, chicken and fish, and plenty of greens. Use healthy fats, as listed in the "Diet" section. After a week on this diet, gradually add in foods such as those listed under "Ritual Substances, Substitutes, or Counteractive Substances" earlier in this section.

- Supplement. In times of great stress, a Shaman absolutely must consider supplementing his or her diet. Zinc disappears from the body within twenty minutes of an extraordinary stress, which could include the channeling of an otherworldly entity or the performance of a cross-dimensional healing. You need zinc to metabolize B vitamins, known as the stress vitamins. Consider using liquid minerals and vitamins. Women, mix your own liquid fat supplement of equal parts evening primrose oil, black currant oil, and either macadamia nut, flaxseed, cranberry, or avocado oil, under the guidance of a natural physician. Men, consider using flaxseed, cranberry, avocado, and evening primrose oil, as well as macadamia nut oil.

- Protect. To protect your life energy and integrity, develop a veneer or energetic protection that keeps harmful energies or entities outside your body. Consider visualizing rose, gold, or white energies around your entire body; if you receive messages from many negative entities, protect with silver and black energies.

- Journey inward. Shamans are able to journey through worlds. Traveling as a soul while leaving the body can leave you susceptible to entity invasion. All worlds are available inside the self.

Style: What does a Shaman look like? Either like a shaman, or, conversely, not like a shaman! Most indigenous Shamans dress the part, understanding that a little flair, a lot of color, and a bold finish induce awe in their patients and community. A "berserk" look can convince the most questioning of clients that the Shaman is a force to be reckoned with. The more powerful a patient perceives the Shaman to be, the more apt the patient is to recover. This perception carries into the spiritual realm. An authoritative appearance scares negative entities. Hence, Shamans are known for wearing flowing frocks, feathers and rocks, and other wild clothing. If you desire this type of shamanic power, develop a style that cultivates a magical and mysterious appearance.

Other Shamans prefer to hide their powers and gifts under the cloak of normalcy. After all, Shamans are contrary, sometimes even in relation to the rest of their caste! If you are a Shaman, know that you can achieve a mystique without looking like mayhem, but consider ways to disguise the tools that offer your body protection. Stone energies are available even if the stones are set in an eighteen-carat gold band. A fancy, signature umbrella can be a wand in disguise. Think through each of your accessories and choose those that have a "magical" alter ego.

Supportive Assistants:

- Mentors. The indigenous Shaman spends years apprenticing with older and wiser elders. If you have been newly introduced to your ability, ask the Divine for a living mentor, and judge this candidate by the health of his or her physical body and the balance maintained among relationships, work, and play.
- Guides. All Shamans work with invisible guides. Ask the Divine to appoint you the correct otherworldly teachers, particularly

ones who will support you in achieving optimum health. My book *Advanced Chakra Healing* describes many such beings.

- A dream guide. Shamans frequently receive revelation through dreams, whether at night or when awake. Ask the Divine to appoint you a dream guide to bring you the dreams and interpretations that will support you in your quest for a perfect body.
- The higher self. We all have a wiser, more mature self. Call upon your own higher self for insight and revelation.

Chakra Nine: Idealist

Spiritual Motivation: When children are starving elsewhere in the world, an Idealist sometimes believes that he or she must also go hungry. To overcome the tendency to disregard your own needs, consider that you can serve more people and help more of humanity if you are healthy.

Endocrine Effects: The diaphragm isn't actually an endocrine organ, but it is a major player in the endocrine system, regulating the breath and therefore the availability of oxygen in the body. The word for breath in Greek, Hebrew, and Latin is the same as the word for "spirit." By improving the influence of your breath in your body, you are vitalizing your body and soul for good work.

Diet: The color of the Idealist's psychic world is gold, the energy of practical miracles. You will seldom find an overweight Idealist; most of them simply forget to eat. The first rule for the Idealist, then, is to remember to eat. Enjoy at least one major meal a day, grazing in between. Consider formulating a diet plan based on your culture or ethnicity, selecting the best and healthiest foods of a particular group as your focus. In general, foods healthy for the third and fourth chakras are best for you.

Exercise: Busy helping others, you can forget that your own body has needs. Base your exercise on the breath. Try yoga, the martial arts, Qigong, tai chi, walking, or even Tae-Bo. You would benefit from weight lifting, which encourages correct breathing, to increase your muscle mass.

Pitfalls and False Pleasures:
- Undereating. Your body needs fuel. Fill it.
- Malnutrition. You can exist for years with a nutritional deficit or a lack of self-care, and you often do. But, bottom line, you can't help anyone else if you aren't helping yourself.
- Physical challenges. Gold extends from the yellow of the third chakra and is the highest potential color of the heart. Thus, your physical ailments duplicate those affecting Thinkers and Relaters. Unusual sensitivities can include precious metals like gold, platinum, or titanium; heavy metals; and planetary or universal energies. Many Idealists also react to events negatively affecting people in other countries, as well as beliefs adversely affecting other cultures. They can also sense and are affected by communal or countrywide curses, miasms (energetic structures that hold people in a negative illness pattern, such as AIDS, or mental structure, such as victimization), and environmental hazards, such as the devastation caused by tsunamis, earthquakes, or violent storms.
- A weak aura. Idealists often have weak ninth auric fields, unconsciously thinning this field in order to take in someone else's problems and help him or her. This absorbed energy overloads the Idealist's body with others' illnesses and issues and compromises the magnetic frequencies of all auric fields. Weak magnetism invites further physical illness, and it inhibits the ability to magnetize or manifest personal needs. This could be why so many Idealists are victims of poverty, a poor constitution, anemia, infertility, and unfulfilling relationships.

Success Tips:
- Breath work. Use your diaphragm! Consider this simple technique for release and manifestation. Inhale and hold your breath for four seconds, during which time you state internally what you want to release or allow the Divine to take. Now exhale. At the end of the exhalation, decide what you desire to magnetize or

allow the Divine to bring to you. Use this process to release old patterns and attract sustenance.

- Draw blood. Idealists are often sensitive to the issues of their ancestors. Make this work for you by constructing a perfect body plan by bloodline. Consider your ethnic, cultural, or spiritual roots. Which diets, health techniques, and philosophies kept your ancestors in optimum shape? By following a similar regime, you invite forward your perfect body and ancestors to support your process.
- Eat. Review the "Diet" section. If you are really challenged by guilt about world hunger, pledge a certain amount of your monthly food budget to adopt a child in another country. Then eat.
- Supplementation. Idealists can tend toward anemia and low blood sugar. If you do, consider taking inositol, magnesium, potassium, zinc with B vitamins, and iron, under the care of a natural physician.
- Complementary supplementation. Idealists with physical maladies frequently respond well to out-of-the-ordinary care, such as homeopathic remedies and tinctures of silver, gold, frankincense, and myrrh.
- Auric supplementation. Every morning, thicken your auric field by interlacing strands of gold throughout every layer. This will compensate for your too-open nature and invite spiritual energies into your body that will help you and others without a strain on your system.
- Transmission. The number one way Idealists learn is through transmission, the acceptance of psychic energy from higher sources. Transmit your perfect body plan from a trusted source or holy person, as well as the advice and energies needed daily to follow it.

Style: Idealists are most comfortable when their clothing, home décor, or belongings reflect a cause. Mold your personal style around your primary soul purpose or life cause, and then customize your environment to match your spiritual values. Many an Idealist selects a favorite culture or ethnicity to represent his or her true spirit.

Supportive Assistants:
- A swami. Idealists often relate to holy men and women. Consider receiving mentorship from a guru, swami, master, or spiritual leader. Note, however, that most holy persons tend to exist on "air," and seldom move except to meditate in a new stance. Select a spiritual mentor who understands the basic needs and beauty of the body.
- A breath coach. Breath cleanses and manifests. Hire someone to help you use your breath to discard physical and psychic waste and open to life's abundant flow of love.
- A friend. Some of the best "breath work" involves talking—or crying or laughing. Of all the chakra types, you are the most susceptible to thinking that spiritual beings do not need human inspiration. When establishing a perfect body plan, ask a friend to partner with you. Review all your accomplishments daily with your companion, and make sure that you share your feelings.

Chakra Ten: Naturalist

Spiritual Motivation: You know that your spiritual mission is to support the world of Nature, so what better way to aid Nature than to call forth your natural self? Your perfect body will most easily emerge if persuaded by a Nature-based protocol, food, and supports. Chemical sprays and processed diet foods are not for you.

Endocrine Effects: The bones carry key life material, including DNA, RNA, ancestral experiences, and soul memories. Naturalists are especially influenced by their bones and the energies that affect the bones.

Bone cells are made of silicon, which are crystals. Crystal cells are receptor cells, and they gather and transmit both sensory and psychic information. These cells attune to the songs of the planet and the stars. When aligned, these crystals structure the body in alliance with the energies of the physical universe. Thus, Naturalists are exceptionally sensitive to the movement, functions, and bodies of the environment. To quicken the emergence of your perfect body, you must attune to the natural cycles of the planets, moon, seas, seasons, and earth.

Your bones demand that you support your perfect body with natural products. Respect the natural processes of your body. Eat when you are hungry, and sleep when you are tired. Flowing with your inherent rhythm invites integration of your subconscious, unconscious, and higher consciousness deep within your bone marrow, which contains the genetic and energetic codes for your ideal body. Bone marrow produces blood cells; you can literally alter your blood, bloodline, and genetic programs by devoting yourself to the power of Nature. This alchemy is yours to choose. To benefit from your inner nature, know that Nature does not dictate your life decisions. You do.

Diet: As a Naturalist, your body is extraordinarily sensitive to chemical additives, pollutants, and antibiotics. Follow these pointers for a nourishing diet:

- Eliminate processed foods. Cut out white flour and sugars, artificially manufactured foods, additives, and chemicals.
- Buy fresh fruits and vegetables.
- Eat organic. Look at labels and choose foods that are not only organic but also free of chemical additives. Avoid smoked or sugared meats and nitrates.
- Think of the earth. Naturalists' main foods are produced in soil. Go with whole grains, oatmeal, brown rice, nuts, potatoes, squash, pumpkin, and other complex carbohydrates, avoiding pasta and white rice. Enjoy fresh or frozen fruits and vegetables, and if you consume dairy, look for farm-fresh dairy products.
- Use spices sparingly. Avoid table salt as much as possible, and liven your meal with fresh herbs and spices.
- Consider vegetarianism. Many Naturalists prefer the vegetarian or vegan lifestyle. Animals are your friends. If you eat meat, consider eating seafood and poultry instead of red meat.

Exercise: Most Naturalists in touch with their inner selves don't have to worry about exercise because they are too busy moving. Whether it is hiking at dawn, chopping wood, or cooking an organic dinner for family and companion animals, Naturalists perform their life activities with physical intensity and fluidity. If stuck inside or in an office, do whatever is necessary to go outside as often as possible. Just walking is enough if done outdoors.

Pitfalls and False Pleasures:

- Allergies. Many Naturalists are actually allergic to inorganic or artificial foods, materials, or substances. Ironically, Naturalists are also frequently affected by natural allergies, such as to dust, animals, and pollen. Test for allergies if you seem sensitive and consider natural treatments including homeopathy, changes in diet, and locally grown honey for airborne allergies.
- Physical maladies. Naturalists are most susceptible to diseases like bone and blood disorders, genetic problems, and environmental sensitivities. The latter can include oversensitivity to planetary or earth changes, weather or climatic shifts, electromagnetic earth energies, power lines, natural and human-created radiation, and other toxic or biological elements.
- Extreme environmentalism. Some Naturalists work themselves into an emotional or a physical frenzy because of their attunement to Nature and the feelings and needs of animals and plants. Unfortunately, living completely naturally—and expecting others to do the same—is not possible. Your environmental efforts must be a realistic endeavor or the strain of perfectionism will cause health crises.
- Ancestral exposure. Grounded in the tenth chakra, which lies beneath the earth, Naturalists are the most able to draw earth energy into themselves. They are also most susceptible to genetic, energetic, and ghostly interference or "hauntings." Through the DNA in their genes, Naturalists can be infected by the illnesses, energies, problems, patterns, and actual energies of those that lived before them. These interfering energies can block the unfolding of the perfect body, prevent the absorption of natural and supernatural energies needed to develop this body, and cause mental and emotional challenges.

Success Tips:

- Join a food co-op. It is cheaper and healthier to shop at a whole foods co-op for food and supplements.

- Eat for your type. Many Naturalists benefit by developing a diet plan based on one of these three ideas: eating for blood type, ethnicity, or locality. Naturalists respond best to foods that match their own genetics and their environmental surroundings.
- Go natural when possible. Eat and dress naturally and organically. Use natural supplements and fill your house with items from the outdoors. Put a fountain in your bedroom to cleanse yourself of the day's stress, and learn which rocks, crystals, natural implements, plants, and energies produce which effects inside and outside of you. Nature is your teacher; watch and learn from her.
- Substitute for health. If you are allergic or reactive to any chemical or natural substances, consider natural substitutes. Try soy or rice milk instead of cow's milk, or carob powder instead of chocolate.
- Natural remedies. Naturalists typically respond best to natural treatments, including herbs, vitamin, and mineral supplementation; magnetic or light therapies; crystal or rock therapies; colonics and detoxification procedures; and the use of poultices, tinctures, and aromatherapies. Aromatherapy, the use of scents and oils, can clear up anything from stress to an emotional or even physical heart wound in many Naturalists.
- Clear out the clutter. Too much dirt, dust, pesticides, or chemicals will derail the Naturalist, as will a home full of muddle and jumble. Use ionic air purifiers, charcoal water purifiers, hypoallergenic pillows or blankets, or other products to keep your nose clear. And organize, organize, organize. Pitch out old papers and clothes and anything else that causes disorder.
- Type your issues. Tenth-chakra individuals can sometimes benefit from this unusual diagnostic technique. Your external environment often reflects your inner reality and vice versa. Have problems with the plumbing? Look for an issue in your colon. Did lightning strike your roof? Perhaps you have been avoiding a seventh-chakra spiritual revelation.
- Desensitization. If you are sensitive to any substance, try desensitization. Clean out your house, system, or body of the potentially troublesome substance and then very gradually add it back. Through

this method you will determine your problematic substance, as well as your breaking point.

- Adventure travel. Many Naturalists lose weight and transform into healthier versions of themselves during vacation, as long as these holidays are spent outdoors. If at all possible, spend your vacation time in nature.
- Break the DNA chain. Naturalists are often susceptible to physical or psychic DNA disturbances. Besides the scientifically validated genetic disorders, you can also inherit issues from ancestors, from your own soul, and through negative bonds to external entities. If you think that you might be affected by any type of genetic problem, you might first work with a professional to determine the root of your disorder. You're trying to find out if the disturbance is physical or psychic, organic or spiritual, from inside or outside of you. Look for qualified and sensitive holistic practitioners, spiritual advisors, or a pastor, priest, or rabbi.
- Work etherically. The tenth auric field surrounds the skin and is often called the etheric field. Learn about techniques for working with it and the etheric mirror, an energy body related to this field, to change your energetic and genetic DNA and clear physical issues. My book *Advanced Chakra Healing* describes this body and healing processes to use. Picture yourself running gold and pink energy throughout this field daily to cleanse and purify it and to enhance your perfect body.

Style: Naturalists by nature appear, well, natural! There is not a polyester shirt in a Naturalist's closet, nor anything but cotton underwear in his or her dresser drawer. Naturalists always appear unaffected and unpretentious. Comfortable in their own skins, they like the feel and texture of natural fabrics and organic materials, and they glow as a result of natural lotions and body products. Dressed in the most breathable clothing in colors that mirror those of the earth and stars, and wearing accessories forged from the earth's materials, the Naturalist will sigh in relief.

Supportive Assistants:

- Natural physicians and practitioners. Consider chiropractors, acupuncturists, holistic counselors, shamans, energy or vibrational healers, homoeopathists, body workers, naturopaths, and nutritionists to help you create your diet, exercise, and healing plans.
- A trail guide. Think of creating your perfect body as the cutting of a path through a forest. Now hire a "trail guide," someone to assist, advise, and cheer you on.
- A spa. Most spas have been transformed into healing havens of holistic care. Whether located in the desert, mountains, or an urban hotel, they can often provide a good start and the education necessary to assist the Naturalist in perfecting his or her body.
- A feng shui master. A Naturalist's home absolutely must support his or her body goals. Consider hiring a feng shui advisor or the equivalent to adjust your home to help you achieve your goals.
- Natural spirit guides. Since the beginning of time, knowledgeable individuals in indigenous communities have turned to the spirits of Nature for protection, insight, and teaching. Ask the Divine to show you which natural guides have been matched to you, and how they can assist you. Consider reading books like *Animal Speak* by Ted Andrews (Llewellyn Publications) if you are working with animal guides.
- Ancestral helpers. Your ancestors can carry hurtful elements, but members of your clan can also help you. Cultures including the Mayan, Native American, East Indian, Chinese, Hmong, Australian aboriginal, Japanese, and dozens of others conduct ceremonies to draw upon the wisdom and assistance of their forebears.

Chakra Eleven: Commander

Spiritual Motivation: The Commander is born to lead. You will be motivated to bring forth your perfect body if you think of your body as an instrument for your powerful personality. To be in charge of others you must take charge of yourself.

Endocrine Effects: How can connective tissue be considered an endocrine gland? Connective tissue supports and surrounds organs and other body parts. It is made of collagen, elastic and reticular fibers, fatty tissue, and cartilage or bone. Granted, this tissue is more affected by hormones than being the producer of them, yet it contains the chemicals key to a Commander's performance and health.

Commanders connect. Leadership is a matter of linking people to address a cause, encouraging them to follow an ethical ideal. The body's connective tissue has this same job, attaching cells and organs to allow fluid and goal-oriented motion. A Commander's perfect body has to display the same characteristics; most Commanders are strong yet physically flexible, and can often appear robust. Commanders must present a robust presence to encourage connection.

Diet: The foods that fuel a Commander's perfect body are those that encourage healthy hormone production and invite detoxification of pollutants and wastes. Avoid chemical-laden foods, and meats and dairy with hormones and antibiotics. Refrain from white flour, white sugar, alcohol, cow's milk products, and foods with MSG, nitrates, and chemical preservatives. Buy products made with omega-3 fatty acids, like olive oil, which support the health of your liver and connective tissue. Fuel your muscles and tissues with high-protein foods, loads of water and tea, whole grains, and lots of fruit and vegetables.

Exercise: A Commander must do full-body exercise as well as exercises for specific parts of the body. Take advantage of your competitive nature and join a sports team. This will file the edge off your tendency to operate in fast-forward and get your body in peak condition. You will train and stay in shape because you do not want to let down your teammates. Then lift weights and try Pilates or some other stretching exercise. You have to work each joint and muscle in the body, because you excel mentally and physically when your connective tissues are in shape.

Pitfalls and False Pleasures:
- Depression. This is not biological depression, but instead the self-denigration that occurs if a Commander is not able to flex his or her leadership muscles. Without a purpose, a Commander

deflates like a balloon lacking air. Find your purpose and you will be happy.

- Grandiosity. Some Commanders struggle with egotism, the belief that being a leader makes them better than others. This grand thinking inhibits intimacy and leads to loneliness. Your perfect body might be "hard" on the outside, but remember to stay "soft" on the inside.
- Bossiness. If you lack humility you won't listen to the advice of those who can help you with your perfect body plan.
- Negativity. As a Commander, you have an inherent ability to transform negative energies into positive energies. If you do not take charge of this psychic gift, however, you will become overwhelmed with negativity and depression.
- Overeating. The stress of being in charge can lead to compulsive eating. Naturally strong and healthy, you are also often hungry and can gravitate toward fatty foods and meats, even choosing "health foods" that are too high in calories.
- Physical challenges. The Commander is vulnerable to problems with connective tissues and muscles, arthritis, bursitis, early aging, and overextension addictions, such as drinking, eating, exercising, or working too much.
- Sensitivities. Most Commanders are sensitive to others' dark or depressive moods, as well as to changes in climate, planetary, and earth energies. Connective tissues link physical and psychic energies. Able to convert natural and human energies into power, Commanders can harness good or bad forces for higher ends, if they are properly trained.

Success Tips:
- Be square. You require lots of fuel to keep moving. Avoid the tendency to overeat, however, by eating three meals a day with protein at each meal; meals should be heavier on the carbohydrates in the morning than in the evening. Drink tea and water between meals.

- Stretch. Your chakra type tends toward bulkiness. Strength is great, but fluidity is also important for your mind-set and as an antiaging strategy. Consider stretching before and after exercising.
- Propel your perfect body plan with boot camp. With your doctor's permission, start strong, as if entering the military. Join a club, select a trainer, set your goals, and go!
- Love. Your strong leadership attributes can scare others and convince you that you do not need love. Open your heart. The key to transforming negativity into positive power lies in your ability to see and treat yourself and others with compassion.
- Say "no." Commanders are such good leaders that everyone wants to put them in charge. Chairing every committee or fund-raiser can leave you drained and vulnerable to the deficiencies of this chakra type, such as overeating or depression. Learn to say "no."

Style: Commanders simultaneously draw attention to themselves while deferring to rank. Wearing a uniform accomplishes these goals and provides credibility as a leader. You don't need to dress in an official uniform (although a great number of Commanders do fill the ranks of uniformed officers), but you will look and feel your best if clothed in your own version of a uniform. When shopping, select clothing of a similar cut, coloring, and feel. You will engender trust from those around you, and you will encourage the pride that enables you to follow a perfect body program.

Supportive Assistants:
- A living mentor. Which leaders exhibit the attributes you also display? Select a mentor and get advice.
- A deceased mentor. Look to the past and create a "board of directors" of those you admire. Have weekly meetings in your imagination with this fellowship, assigning the board the task of helping you develop and live your perfect body and life.
- A master. Every religious order has mentors, whether they are Jesus or the saints, masters and avatars, or prophets and seers. Select a master as your personal guide for physical and spiritual development.

5

Perfecting Your Perfect Body Plan

*You see, Wendy, when the first baby laughed for
the first time, its laugh broke into a thousand pieces,
and they all went skipping about, and that was the
beginning of fairies. And now, whenever a new
baby is born, its first laugh becomes a fairy.*

J.M. Barrie, *Peter Pan*

In his classic children's tale *Peter Pan*, master storyteller J. M. Barrie claims that fairies first splintered from the laugh of a baby. As each fairy carries reverberations of a baby's laughter, so does each of us mirror the characteristics of the Divine, the parent of us all. As a child of the Creator, you can also create what you really desire, including your perfect body.

It is time to construct your perfect body plan from your knowledge of your strongest chakra traits. This plan will be the culmination of the information that you have gathered so far. It will also assist you in structuring your actions and attitudes until you achieve your ideal life.

To write your plan, begin by reviewing the exercise and narrative that you completed at the end of chapter 3. What kind of person are you? What are your core strengths, weaknesses, and needs? Now add this assessment to the information in chapter 4, selecting the chakra configurations that reflect your strongest chakras. If you have one strong chakra, read through the description of that chakra in relation to your perfect body. If you have more than one strong chakra, it will be necessary to consider the characteristics of each chakra type and blend them into a unified whole.

In this chapter I share examples of client plans, stories of clients who followed those plans, and questions to help you formulate your own perfect body plan. By the end of this chapter you will have produced an outline that you can use to attract your perfect body. Remember to have fun with this process. If the fairies emerged from a single laugh, image the divine chuckle that birthed the rest of us!

This section provides two types of examples to help you create your own perfect body plan. First, I offer three case studies of people with one, two, and three strong chakras. These stories will show you the depth to which you can go when you are working with your plan. Second, I provide samples of four actual plans. These are based on chakra personality configurations involving four strong chakras, more than four strong chakras, all mid-range scores, and all weak scores. These examples will show you what a perfect body plan can look like. Finally, you will be ready to develop your own customized plan using the provided questions.

Each plan covers the following categories:
- Spiritual Motivation
- Endocrine Effects
- Diet
- Exercise
- Pitfalls and False Pleasures
- Success Tips
- Style
- Supportive Assistants

PLANNING FOR SUCCESS: STORIES OF REAL PEOPLE

Configuration One: If You Have One Strong Chakra

Having a single strength makes your job easy. You only have to review one of the chakra personality profiles from chapter 4 to construct your plan. The challenge is to compensate for the weaknesses inherent in each chakra personality, for which I recommend tapping into the strengths of at least one supportive chakra. Let us look at how one of my single-chakra clients created his perfect body plan in order to assist you in creating your own.

Charles was the consummate first-chakra personality. He had grown his home-based business into a giant retail business with dozens of stores nationwide. Working up to eighteen hours a day, he made no time for relationships or play. Then he had a heart attack. At age forty-four, Charles now yearned for a new life, starting with a healthy body.

Charles and I started by developing a brief perfect body plan based on his first-chakra Manifester traits. We also drew upon his secondary gifts from his seventh Spiritual chakra. Here are the highlights.

Spiritual Motivation: A spiritual man, Charles believed that God had given him his business for a greater purpose. People needed the products that he provided through his stores. Charles therefore reasoned that better health would enable him to better serve his retail clients, and therefore serve God.

Endocrine Effects: After reading the summary description of an adrenal-based person, Charles laughed. "That is me, exactly!" he said. To uncover his perfect body, he vowed to maintain a healthier balance of work, play, and relationships, with his cardiologist's advice.

Diet: Charles created a diet plan based on four factors: his cardiologist's recommendations; advice from a naturopath; the foods best suited to an adrenal-based person; and the heart-healthy recommendations listed for fourth-chakra personalities. We reviewed the latter list because he had already suffered a heart attack.

To support his adrenal personality, Charles agreed to eat three meals a day, to take the appropriate supplements, and to drink ten glasses of water daily. His basic diet consisted of high-fiber grains, grass-fed beef and organic poultry, and lots of vegetables.

Charles reluctantly eliminated sugar, hard alcohol, and almost all white flour, and he added to his diet supplements for his heart, including CoQ10, folic acid, a glass of red grape juice daily, decaffeinated black and green teas, and extra omega-3 fatty acids, including flaxseed oil. He also added adrenal supports, including vitamins B and C with a zinc tablet in the morning, extra vitamin B_5, and extra water.

For cooking, he used grapeseed or olive oil, and he added lots of heart-healthy spices like cayenne pepper, turmeric, garlic, and onion. Snack foods included walnuts (rich in omega-3 fatty acids), real fruit yogurt, vegetables, and apples. I also encouraged Charles to eat plenty of white fish, especially if ordering dinner at a restaurant, which is helpful for the pineal gland, the major organ of his supportive seventh chakra.

Exercise: Charles set up a graduated exercise plan with a physical therapist recommended by his cardiologist, working his first- and seventh-chakra needs into his program. He walked daily. To accentuate his Spiritualist abilities, I taught him how to enfold prayer and meditation into his walking time. He joined a yoga group, thus releasing adrenal stress while enjoying the Spiritualist's desire for contemplation; and he started weight lifting, a usual "must" for hard-driving Manifesters.

Pitfalls and False Pleasures: Both Charles and I were clear about his potential challenges, which fell into three categories: work, intimacy, and sleep. Orphaned at a young age, Charles learned not to trust relationships; work was a seemingly valid excuse for avoiding friendships and a spouse. His fear of intimacy created a sort of self-alienation. Afraid to be alone unless working, Charles seldom went to bed before midnight. There he tossed and turned, only sleeping a few hours before rising at dawn to do guess what? Work! A heart cannot heal without sleep; neither is a life fruitful without love. Charles also guessed that as soon as he started feeling fit, he would think that he was healthy again and would taper off his perfect body regimen.

Success Tips: We put these strategies into place to avoid potential pitfalls.

1. For overwork: We scheduled Charles's walk for the middle of the day, right before lunch, so he had a prolonged break. We then planned weight lifting for 8 A.M. three times a week, so he did not have to rise before 7 A.M. on those days. He also signed up for yoga twice a week at 6 P.M., assuring that he left work by 5 P.M. on those days. Next, we teamed up with his secretary and prebooked four vacations for the next year. She then promised to book an in-office therapeutic massage with a Shiatsu expert once a week. Charles agreed to allow his secretary to keep him on his "health schedule" and book meetings around these appointments.
2. For intimacy: We drew upon Charles's Spiritualist characteristics and he joined a church and its singles' group.
3. For sleep: Charles agreed upon a bedtime of 10 P.M., except for nights when he had his singles' group. Adrenal types must have a reward. Charles's reward was that he could read an adventure novel for half an hour when in bed. We also revamped Charles's bedroom to make it conducive to sleep. A feng shui expert eliminated all vestiges of work and placed a waterfall and appropriate stones, crystals, and candles in his bedroom. His naturopath also gave him valerian, a natural sleep aid, for those restless nights.

Style: To reflect his current success, Charles engaged the services of a personal shopping assistant to help him choose an appropriate wardrobe. She went with him to a well-known clothier, a source for quality clothes for work, play, and home. She then introduced him to the concept of having those clothes tailored to fit him perfectly.

Supportive Assistants: We created a team of assistants around Charles. Because Manifesters are concrete, most of his assistants were "real," not spirit-based, and included his cardiologist, a naturopath, his secretary, a physical therapist, a personal shopping assistant, a feng shui expert, and a massage therapist. He also began to use the pastor through his church and the singles' group for spiritual guidance, and he considered me to be his spiritual and emotional life coach. At my recommendation, Charles also established an invisible "board of directors," consisting of his heroes and spiritual mentors, with whom he would consult about business problems.

Outcome: One year later, Charles was thirty pounds lighter, robust, toned—and dating a woman he had met in his singles' group! She had three children, which forced him into leisure activities. His cardiologist was amazed at his health progress, and despite brief relapses into overwork and a liking for frosting-covered cinnamon rolls, Charles was easily able to stick to his diet and his exercise plan.

Configuration Two: If You Have Two Strong Chakras

If you have two equally strong chakras you can use ideas from each, depending upon which profile is more appropriate at the moment. Of course, it is more effective to consult both sets of chakra traits right from the start, as did Darla, a Feeler-Naturalist.

Darla had one goal: losing weight. She had an uncontrollable urge to consume anything in sight that was white. Cookies, donuts, muffins, bread. . . the temptations were numerous, and she succumbed to them all.

Darla's stressors included four children, a full-time job, and a farm. Married to a farmer, Darla frequently assisted him with the dairy cows and an overabundance of chores. Depressed about her weight, she hid behind thick glasses and drab housedresses and just kept "plowing ahead," as she put it.

I determined almost immediately that Darla was victim to a typical Feeler malady, candida. To verify this, I sent her to a holistic medical doctor for tests; the doctor confirmed my diagnosis. Given her Naturalist profile, she was probably sensitive if not allergic to most chemically processed foods.

Darla wanted a simple plan, so we created the following basic blueprint.

Spiritual Motivation: Darla wanted to feel happier and show her natural beauty. She decided that God wanted her to be healthier as a way of assuring both goals.

Endocrine Effects: As a Feeler, Darla was affected by her hormones, particularly her ovaries. Like many Feelers with candida, she experienced severe premenstrual syndrome (PMS). As a Naturalist, her well-being was also influenced by her bones, which determine bodily structure and the production of blood cells. We therefore needed to better support her hormonal health, as well as her basic body structure.

Diet: Though she wanted to lose weight, Darla did not really want to diet. So I simply advised her to refrain from eating any white food. With this one step, we eliminated the foods nourishing the candida and those foods containing the greatest number of chemical additives. To provide extra minerals and good fats, she prescribed to the liquid supplement program I describe in the appendix (see page 136). Darla also agreed to drink eight glasses of water a day, in addition to using white and green teas for a taste treat, and to supplement her diet with extra antioxidants.

Exercise: Despite her hectic schedule, Darla seldom increased her heart rate, so I suggested that she select two exercises. As a Naturalist, she agreed to walk outside for thirty minutes every evening after work. This would also give her a much-needed break from tending to everyone else's problems. She engaged a friend as a walking companion, a helpful trick for a Feeler. The two of them agreed to help each other by listening to what feelings had arisen that day for each of them. In this way, Darla learned to let go of her emotional stress in a healthy way, a major accomplishment for a Feeler.

Darla next agreed to swim twice a week at the high school, where she was employed as a teacher. Feelers are natural swimmers, and water invites emotional release, also washing others' feelings from the body. Darla also agreed to recite the phrase "I am now releasing others' feelings and needs" when swimming laps as part of her perfect body program.

Pitfalls and False Pleasures: Darla's main challenges centered on her entrenched pattern of taking care of others' needs and feelings instead of her own. Her habit of taking second place in her own life, as well as her dietary dysfunctions, could topple her entire program.

Success Tips: First, Darla needed to establish her own sacred space. Feelers are constantly confronted by others' feelings and issues, and they absolutely must spend time alone to compensate. After arguing that there were no extra rooms in her house for her to use, Darla selected a corner in their four-season porch, using a screen for privacy. She followed her Naturalist urgings to decorate the space, filling it with rocks, feathers, logs, and other objects found on her walks. After a while, she started stapling scraps of colorful fabric on the walls, drawing upon her creative Feeler gifts to create an art space. On her own, Darla purchased a tai chi tape and began to do tai chi at dawn in this space, gaining a peace of mind that carried her through the day.

Second, Darla agreed to spend half an hour with her husband in their bedroom every night. Feelers are sensual creatures, and their perfect bodies often need to be invited forth with touch, taste, and laughter. After a few months of sharing this time with her husband, Darla took a massage class and introduced her husband to the joys of massage with aromatic oils. Needless to say, these shared times began to be a highlight of both their days!

Third, Darla consulted with a BioSET professional, using this computer-based methodology to clear up her food allergies (see page

136 for additional information on BioSET). Her cravings were cut in half, and she was easily able to maintain her diet after eight sessions. When she did "cheat," she did not succumb to days of binge eating; instead, she climbed right back on her diet wagon.

Style: Darla did not understand why she had to dress differently *before* losing weight. I pointed out that self-care is an important part of developing one's perfect body. Wearing clothes and colors associated with one's inner spirit actually entices the emergence of a Feeler's ideal body, and establishing an appropriate environment encourages the Naturalist. Not quite convinced by my reasoning, Darla agreed to buy three outfits, consisting of two pairs of stretch cotton pants (which would adapt to her forthcoming weight loss), and a pair of black silk pants. She then bought three long silk shirts of various gemstone colors; Feelers are creative, and they feel happiest when dressed originally and colorfully. I suggested she select hues that she believed reflected her true nature. Finally, we added accessories of stones associated with Naturalist and Feeler attributes, which Darla reported seemed "particularly energizing." After a day at the hair stylist, Darla was a new woman!

Supportive Assistants: As already mentioned, Darla used a holistic medical doctor for developing her diet and engaged a friend as an exercise partner and an emotional sounding board. The BioSET practitioner and I rounded out her initial team.

As time went on, we added three more assistants. First we engaged a makeup artist who taught Darla how to buy and apply organic-based makeup. Second, Darla began working with a holistic chiropractor, thus helping her bones and posture as well as relieving her stress. Finally, Darla attended a seminar on Native American power animals, and in meditation she met the guiding spirit of a bear, who helped her stay strong when she was tempted to return to her old ways of eating white food and caretaking her family.

Outcome: One year later, Darla was a trim, voluptuous 160 pounds, down from 202 pounds. She continued to follow her diet and exercise protocol, but had cut her work to part-time. She and her husband had so enjoyed their extra time together that they decided it would be best to have Darla help more with the farming business. Darla decided to continue her supplements after the one-year mark. The eyeglasses were gone, and so were the housedresses. Darla now dressed almost exclusively in cotton and silk; she went to the hairdresser every week; and she looked ten years younger than she had just a year before! Her artistic inclinations had been transferred from her sacred space into the remainder of the home, which is now a den of bright colors and interesting textures.

Configuration Three: If You Have Three Strong Chakras

With three strong chakras, you have an abundance of assets to draw upon. Organize your strengths and you can attain that perfect body in no time!

How do you best construct a perfect body plan given your diverse needs and strengths? Start by imagining an equilateral triangle. All sides are equal, as are your chakric abilities and needs. To make your plan, stand in the middle and choose a little of this chakra and a little of that one until you are pleased with the results.

Fred, for example, was a Thinker, Idealist, and Naturalist. Scrawny, which is typical of all three body types, he compulsively worried about every aspect of eating, including food composition, world hunger ethics, and pricing value. "The problem is, I'm down to almost no foods," he complained. "Take nuts. Peanuts have mold, cashews are too expensive, and though soy beans are healthy, how can I eat up some of the world's available soy resources when . . ."

I finished Fred's sentence for him. "There are starving children that don't have enough food?"

He blinked. "Yes."

Fred exhibited characteristics from all three chakras. As a Thinker, he relished a structured, logical, and inexpensive health care regime. An Idealist, he wanted assurance that his health would not cost others their health. Like most Naturalists, he fretted about the environment, certain that the slightest unnatural substance that entered his mouth or penetrated his skin would cause dire health consequences.

I asked Fred what his "perfect body" would be like. At first he seemed puzzled by the thought, so devoted was he to helping others with their needs, but then he listed characteristics such as a healthier weight, toned muscles, and an assured manner. I showed him the lists associated with each of his strongest chakras and asked whether he could possibly construct a perfect body program from the listed concepts. He seemed relieved. This is what he created.

Spiritual Motivation: Fred agreed that being healthy would enable him to help more people, as long as his process involved actions that aligned with his personal ethics.

Endocrine Effects: As a Thinker, Fred was centered on his solar plexus. He felt every stress in his digestive organs until he was unable to eat. His Naturalist urgings related to his bones, and therefore he needed to select a diet that aligned with his genetic inheritances. Fortunately, this requirement was easily buttressed with his Idealist association with the diaphragm and the related emphasis on selecting foods based on ethical and spiritual ideals. Fred was encouraged by the easy blending of these three glandular types: By creating a perfect body diet and a life plan based on his global idealism, he could use his Thinker planning and organizing skills to develop a daily program that aligned with his Naturalist's environmental sensitivities.

Diet: Fred reviewed the foods suggested in the applicable three categories and then selected the Naturalist's "grazing" diet, choosing to eat five or six small meals a day. This way he could assure himself of a full spectrum of proteins, carbohydrates, and fats and avoid the blood sugar swings sometimes associated with being a Thinker. He selected foods including mercury-free tuna and salmon, mixed nuts, whole-grain crackers, dried fruits, steamed and raw vegetables, hummus, and soy milk and cheese, as all were easy snack foods and aligned with his Naturalist and Idealist belief systems. He already drank lots of water daily, to which we added choices like green and white teas for variety and increased antioxidants.

Exercise: Fred created an exercise program that did not require an expensive gym. Instead, he agreed to walk briskly in a park outfitted with circuit-training resources every day. He could go outside and add brawn at the same time! To tone his body, he selected a number of river rocks, which he agreed to lift every other day while listening to melodic ethnic music.

Pitfalls and False Pleasures: Fred had an inner saboteur, convinced that his own happiness would cost others theirs. As an Idealist, this belief had forced him into a life of near poverty and loneliness. His Naturalist self encouraged malnutrition and emotional and physical oversensitivity. His bright Thinker mind worked against him instead of for him, formulating obsessive-compulsive thoughts that encouraged worry and digestive complaints. We needed to convince Fred that welcoming his perfect body would increase his own and others' happiness so that his Thinker self could support his perfect body protocol.

Success Tips: Fred adopted these techniques to escape his self-sabotage.

1. Grounding. Fred used an important Naturalist method for grounding, linking into the earth as a means to replenish his strength and connect to Nature. He conducted grounding exercises five or six times a day, imaging himself as a tree rooted into the earth.
2. Guidance. During a grounding meditation Fred asked the Great Spirit to appoint him an earth-based guardian spirit. He received an ancestor from his own bloodline and began to check in with this being every morning for life instructions. He also asked this being to help him maintain his "procedures," the term he used for his plan.
3. Supplementing with herbs. Working with a naturopathic friend, Fred supported his dietary changes with natural herbs, a common Naturalist attraction.
4. Cooking ethnically. Fred eventually altered his cooking to use spices and aromatic oils that reflected his ancestry as well as the cultures that interested him. This boosted his Naturalist and Idealist strengths.

5. Writing lists. Fred agreed that his Thinker would benefit by focusing on checklists. Every day Fred wrote a list of "success ideas" and rewarded his Thinker self with a star on the calendar if every item was checked off. A certain number of stars translated into a "cheat treat," usually pecan pie.

Style: At best, Fred's appearance could be described as ragged. We played a game, having him talk to the three main aspects of his chakra personality, a helpful technique when working with multiple chakra types. His Idealist self was allergic to spending money on new clothes when thousands of people do not have them, while the "inner Thinker" thought that Fred would be more effective in his job as a fund-raiser if he looked more dapper. Now the Naturalist piped up, requesting organic cloth. Fred and I examined several magazines and between them selected a look that was fresh, natural, and comfortable yet professional. Fred then shopped for clothing in second-hand stores, which suited his Idealist's ways.

Supportive Assistants: Fred drew upon several visible and invisible forms of support, including the already-mentioned naturopath, a guiding ancestor, and me. A few months later he also added a mentor to help him improve his fund-raising presentations.

Outcome: Fred was amazed at the difference in his physique and psyche at the end of only six months. He was probably proudest of the biceps that bulged (slightly) underneath his all-cotton shirts, but he also bragged about the respectable increase in income he was enjoying due to a more effective fund-raising style. Begrudgingly, he attributed some of the success to his more professional appearance. Fred's eyes teared up when describing his relationship with the earth and his guide, saying that he had always wanted a relationship with the Divine that made sense to him. Now that he had it, he understood the importance of self-care. His newfound interest in herbs was inspiring him to begin working toward a certificate in the field. He hoped to combine this knowledge with his developing culinary skills to start his own natural restaurant one day, one that would feature foods from around the world. With an added ten pounds on his slight frame, Fred looked and felt happy, attractive, and, most important, healthy. In opening to his perfect body, Fred had uncovered his already perfect self.

PLANNING FOR SUCCESS: PLANS BY REAL PEOPLE

Configuration Four: If You Have Four Strong Chakras

The versatility of the four-chakra configuration assures an energized and interesting life. The only trouble is that your varied nature can get you into trouble. Which of your various inner personalities act in accordance with your goals? It is easy to slide into behaviors that defeat bodily health; your gifts are equaled by your weaknesses. If you have four strong chakras, you are going to have to be meticulous and detailed in the creation of a perfect body blueprint.

Tamara had four strong chakras—and an extraordinarily strong personality. She mixed the traits of a fourth-chakra Relater, fifth-chakra Communicator, sixth-chakra Visionary, and eighth-chakra Shaman. Professionally, she had suitably blended her abilities and loved her job as a radio personality, offering relationship coaching during the morning hours when professionals were commuting to work. The only problem was that Tamara, who worked nearly all the time, was fifty pounds overweight. She consumed pots of coffee to be alert after rising at 4 A.M. After her radio spot she pumped herself up with gallons of diet carbonated beverages and ever-present handfuls of donuts, chocolates, and salted nuts. On her big frame, fifty pounds was not overly noticeable, but Tamara also complained of back pain, migraines, exhaustion, and anxiety. She was so miserable that she seldom exercised and never socialized. She wanted a different body, one that would invite enthusiasm for movement and a personal life.

Here is the actual perfect body plan developed by Tamara, written in her own words, along with a summary of the results of following it for six months.

Spiritual Motivation: I want to summon my perfect body so that I can reach my goal of being the top morning commute relationship coach in my region, shamanically transforming the stress of my job into energy for living as the lean, beautiful, powerful person that I really am.

Endocrine Effects: I now picture my heart, thyroid, pituitary, and thymus glands as interconnected, and vow to meet the needs of these four organs by doing activities that coordinate these organs, including:

- Talking on the phone (Communicator) with a friend once a day (Relater), discussing the blessings (Shaman) of my hectic job in relation to my long-range goals (Visionary).
- Getting a hands-on energy healing (Shaman and Relater) from a gifted clairvoyant (Visionary) who can share spiritual insights with me (Communicator).
- Writing insights (Communicator) from my own spiritual guidance (Shaman and Communicator) about my healing needs (Relater) in relation to my long-range perfect body goals (Visionary).

Diet: I choose a heart-based diet, as it is healthiest for my entire body, adding dark chocolate as a reward once a day. This substance will enhance my Visionary skills and curb my sugar cravings. When tired, I will use the list of Shaman substance substitutes, so that I refrain from alcohol, coffee, and sugar, choosing soft but healthy foods to appease my Communicator desires. For supplements, I will add liquid minerals and drink lots of water, as this is recommended for all my strong chakras.

Exercise: I choose to take dancing classes at the Drum Institute after work four times a week. Dancing with others meets my Relater needs; talking to people and listening to the drumming music is a Communicator's dream; dressing in wild dance clothes is enticing for my Visionary self; and drumming itself is a Shaman activity.

Pitfalls and False Pleasures: My biggest temptation is to snack on food at work. After all, everyone else is drinking caffeine and eating do-nuts! In particular, I succumb to cravings because I am so tired, but also because my body hurts in so many places.

Success Tips: To refrain from the buffet of unhealthy food at work, I will tell my coworkers about my perfect body plan and ask for their support. I will request that they start bringing fresh fruit and vege-tables instead of sugary foods, and I will do the same for us all. I will drink caffeinated green tea instead of coffee (I cannot quite give up the energy boost of caffeine), and when I am tempted by a diet car-bonated beverage, I will drink instead a sparkling water flavored with a little heart-healthy grape juice. Spiritually, I will ask the Divine to appoint me a gatekeeper (Shaman), with whom I will speak in med-itation every morning on my way to work (Communicator) (I take the subway, which comprises my only real time alone until evening). I will ask this gatekeeper for advice and support in following my per-fect body program (Relater); in meeting my long-range goals (Vi-sionary); and for protection against negative people and influences (Shaman). I also will schedule hands-on healing with a Matrix Re-patterning expert (see page 137). Matrix repatterning is one of many hands-on healing modalities that can potentially correct my physical and organic disorders.

Style: I must maintain a professional image as a Communicator, but I will now start dressing in comfortable, people-friendly Relater cloth-ing of bright Visionary colors, accessorizing with Shaman-type jew-elry, including crystal necklaces and bracelets.

Supportive Assistants: These are the energies that I am drawing upon to meet my perfect body goals.
- Friends (Relater, Communicator, Visionary, Shaman)
- Dance class members (Relater)
- Coworkers (Relater and Communicator)
- Spiritual gatekeeper (Communicator and Shaman)

• Healers, starting with matrix worker and Cyndi (Relater and Shaman)

Outcome: How did Tamara do? Within six months she had lost twenty of the fifty pounds that she wanted to lose. Three sessions with a Matrix Repatterning expert had eliminated her physical complaints, but they also stimulated several more sessions with me in order to work with the emotions held deep inside. Freeing herself from underlying emotional pains made Tamara a much happier person. Her depression was also alleviated by the emergence of several new friendships; by sharing her vulnerability and engaging with her work fellows, she had struck up friendships with many of them. Professionally, she was now in the process of putting together a new morning commute show on healing, which drew upon her mystical interests, as well as her strengths as a relationship coach. "My life has turned around," shared the attractive, fit, and colorful personality. Like a true Visionary, she then added, "I am not done, but then, life is about the dreams that we still have to achieve, is it not?"

Configuration Five:
If You Have More Than Four Strong Chakras

Do you feel like you are so good at so many things that it is hard to accomplish even the most menial tasks? That is the sentiment shared by James, a five-chakra whiz who was tired of feeling like the "weak kid on the block." At sixteen years of age he looked like a twelve-year-old, and he was tired of being seen as the "little boy" of his high school class. We typed his chakra personality to see whether we could create a simple yet effective perfect body plan.

A straight-A student, James was obviously a Thinker. This attribute was equaled by similar strengths as a Healer, Visionary, Spiritualist, and Idealist. James's life goal was to become a physician and serve abroad as a medical missionary. Thus, his purpose combined elements of all five chakra types, yet he lacked one vital ingredient: self-esteem in relation to his physical appearance. We put this blueprint together. Here it is, in his words.

Spiritual Motivation: I want to develop a muscular and attractive physical presence, so that my peers and authority figures take me more seriously. With greater presence, I can better serve God and humanity as a medical missionary.

Endocrine Effects: I will draw upon my endocrine strengths in order to build muscle mass and assume a "bigger" and more charismatic personality in the world. First, I will find a photograph of my goal body (Visionary) in a white coat (Healer). I will place the photo on the map of a country I want to serve in (Visionary and Idealist), and then daily pray to God for guidance and support to achieve this goal (Spiritualist). I will write down this advice given by God to me on that day and follow it (Thinker).

Diet: I realize that muscles come from protein, but as an Idealist, I have a hard time eating meat when half the world is starving and cannot afford it. I will therefore adopt a fourth-chakra diet, as it reflects the best of all diet types, with these differences:

1. Instead of red meat, I will eat the vegetable and animal proteins of the culture that I eventually want to serve.
2. I will supplement with iron pills, as I am anemic, a fact established by my doctor.
3. I will eat grazing-type meals, concentrating on protein, so that I build muscle mass.
4. I will bless my food. I will give thanks to the animal or fish that gave its life for me, and ask to receive power and strength through its flesh. I will also thank God for the food given to me so that I can better serve Him and humanity.

Exercise: I will combine both cardiovascular and muscle-building exercises, as I understand that these will meet all of my requirements. I choose kickboxing for my aerobic exercise, as it will also build muscle strength and stamina, and I will lift weights at the school gym three times a week. Given that as an Idealist I can prosper from breathing, I will also take a yoga class on the weekends. This relaxation exercise will help my "Thinker self," who has years of stressful study-ing ahead.

Pitfalls and False Pleasures: My greatest weakness is to think that I am nothing but my mind, as getting good grades is how I have forged a reputation for myself. Being religious, I can also tend to disregard the body in favor of spiritual pursuits.

Success Tips: I must apply my Healer philosophy to counterbalance my Spiritualist and Idealist philosophies. Obviously, I care about people's physical health, or I would not want to be a doctor. I will therefore see myself as my own patient. To counteract my mental tendencies, I will apply my Thinker ability to set and establish a plan, as set forth in this program.

Style: In line with my goals, I will start dressing like a successful med-ical missionary, like the person I am becoming. To do this, I will get a briefcase for school that looks like a medical bag; wear at least one item daily that reflects one of the cultures I want to work with; and pray to God for help in showing my inner spirit to the world, as this is the "real self" I want to convey and become.

Supportive Assistants: I promise to use the following to support me:
1. God, through prayer.
2. My parents, who want me to be happy, not just successful. I will tell them my plan.
3. My mom, who can help me with my diet.
4. My friend Jimmy, who is on the football team. He can help me with the weight training.
5. My sister Jane, who is into yoga and all of that "weird stuff." She can take me to a yoga class—if I can convince her not to tell her friends.

Outcome: After writing the plan, James disappeared from my prac-tice. I got a call from him two years later, however, from college. He was pre-med, which was no surprise, but he was also thrilled to report that he had gained twenty pounds in muscle weight, and though still thin and small, he felt robust and attractive. During his last year of high school he started dating one of the popular girls in school, and he ended up starting a yoga group for the football team! I heard from him again a year later. He was still seeing the same young woman and was looking forward to sending me postcards from Bangladesh, where he was going to serve an internship that summer through a mentor, a medical missionary from his church.

Configuration Six:
If Your Chakras Are Mainly in the Mid-range

Many mid-range scorers hide their greatest attribute under a veneer of normalcy. Carla felt safe living in the middle, but she was now tired of being everyone's "plain but nice girl" who never went home with anyone special. Growing up in a chaotic home she had learned to hide her true strengths for fear of the repercussions. About thirty pounds overweight and flabby, with mousy blonde hair, she had suddenly decided to uncover her "real" and beautiful and sexy self.

The first task was to discover Carla's chakra strengths. Discussion illuminated a robust Communicator gift. As a child, Carla had wanted to be a writer, and had exhibited an incredible aptitude. She had also heard spirits speak to her as a child. She shut down both aspects of her fourth chakra in reaction to her parents, who responded with comments like, "You are better off being silent rather than speaking for the devil."

Here is Carla's process. Foremost, we wanted to highlight her Communicator attributes, while engaging the other chakras when necessary.

Spiritual Motivation: I want to express my deepest thoughts and truest self through the development of my perfect body and my communication strengths.

Endocrine Effects: I am willing to see myself as a thyroid-based personality, as long as using fifth-chakra methods of eating and health care cause weight loss. I will get a thyroid panel laboratory blood test from my doctor to see whether I have a medical condition. In addition, I will see a holistic nutritionist to customize my diet. I will then evaluate whether or not I can use my fourth-chakra abilities to establish another career path and to access my psychic gifts.

Diet: I will follow the recommended eating program for a Communicator, as per medical input, adding the basics of the heart-happy Mediterranean diet, as my Relater gifts are slightly more elevated than my other mid-range chakras.

1. I will eat three meals a day.
2. Breakfast shall be either oatmeal or fortified-egg omelets cooked in olive oil, containing steamed vegetables.
3. Lunch will be a green salad with fish or chicken and dark berries or cherries as dessert. I will eat a slice of whole-wheat bread with this meal.
4. Dinner will be fish, chicken, or organic grass-fed beef; steamed vegetables; and a whole-grain carbohydrate. I will eat beets once a week.
5. I will snack on blueberries, cherries, and soup, and I will eat a baked potato before bedtime so I do not snack in the middle of the night. The serotonin in the potato will also help me sleep.
6. I will switch to soy instead of dairy milk (after having seen a holistic nutritionist and being diagnosed as allergic to dairy).
7. I will use liquid supplements, to boost my minerals and heal my body from years of eating too many sweets and breads.

Exercise: I will walk with a friend (as a Relater) three times a week for one hour after work, and walk on my own with musical tapes three other times a week.

False Pleasures and Pitfalls: I am hypothyroid (as the medical lab results revealed; Carla completed several of her blueprint sections after consulting with her doctor and her nutritionist). I think the emotional root of this condition is related to my fear of really expressing myself through speaking, writing, or opening to my psychic abilities. I tend to stay home at night instead of going out, and I hide behind my "bad looks" because I am anxious about being rejected. I am also frightened of switching my career as a secretary, even though I think that I would like public relations, journalism, or another writing-based profession.

Success Tips: To compensate for my fears, I will do the following:
1. Use an acupuncturist to help heal my thyroid.
2. Take the thyroid medication that my doctor prescribes.
3. Join a writer's support group.
4. Research returning to school in journalism and determine whether my company will pay for tuition.
5. Take an intuitive development class from Cyndi, concentrating on using my fifth-chakra gifts.
6. Play Bach at night, to encourage sleep and positive feelings.
7. Ask God to appoint me a gatekeeper, so I feel safe in opening my verbal intuitive abilities.
8. Say "no" at least once a day, and only say "yes" when I really mean it.
9. Wear a necklace with lapis over my throat, to encourage communication.
10. Put an auric screen over the back of my fourth chakra until I am better able to control my verbal psychic gift.

Style: I will go shopping with an intuitive friend and have her help me pick out clothes that match a writer's mentality. I will have her come to the hairdresser and makeup artist with me, to help me discover a new look.

Supportive Assistants: Here are my helpers.
1. Doctor, for the thyroid test.
2. Holistic nutritionist, for the diet.
3. Acupuncturist, to help heal the thyroid problem.
4. Writer's support group.
5. School advisor, for journalism school.
6. Human resource advisor, on my career path and additional schooling.
7. Walking friend.
8. Cyndi and friends met in intuitive development class.

9. Hairdresser and makeup advisor.
10. Gatekeeper, as appointed by God.
11. Licensed therapist (this was added later; see below).

Outcome: After about nine months, Carla published an article in a trade publication on a trip she took to the Amazon. She was ecstatic! By then, she had lost twenty of the thirty pounds that she wanted to lose, and was continuing to see the acupuncturist weekly. After a while, Carla also agreed to see a licensed therapist, uncovering dark secrets from her childhood, which she was still resolving. She had applied and been accepted at the School of Journalism; her employer had agreed to pay for half of the tuition.

Carla and her walking buddy now walked every day, and she had also purchased season tickets to the orchestra; Carla was developing an intense passion for music, and had therefore also signed up for a ballroom dance class. She was also excelling at her intuition classes, and was considering working as an intuitive reader part-time to pay the additional tuition cost for college. Every morning and evening she prayed to the Divine. Her gatekeeper, an angel, provided her inspiration to uphold her perfect body—and life—program. The input included insisting that Carla maintain monthly sessions with her hairdresser! Carla had chosen a blonde hair color offset perfectly by her brighter and more fluid clothes. Carla was now on the path of her perfect life.

Configuration Seven:
If You Have a Lot of Weak Chakras

There is nothing wrong with having weaknesses, as long as you know what your strengths are and use them. Anthony tested nine of eleven chakras as weak, but had two glowing strong chakras, the Commander and the Manifester. I suspected, however, that a few of the lower scoring chakras would rise if he devoted himself to accentuating his strengths, starting with attending to his perfect body.

We started our process with his goal of returning to his college shape in mind. A former college football player, Anthony had continued to eat the vast amounts of food that such a sport allowed, but without doing the exercise that he once did. Here is Anthony's perfect body plan.

Spiritual Motivation: I am an intense kind of guy. I love financially supporting my wife and two girls, but my girth is in my way. No matter how well I dress, people think I am sloppy because my belly hangs over my belt. I am short of breath when climbing the stairs, and get creaky when I try to exercise. I think I am a strong guy, but that God wants me healthier than this so that I can better provide for my family and be around for a long time to come.

Endocrine Effects: I understand that I am an adrenal-based person. I am constantly stressed; I guess that is why I always eat lots of potatoes with gravy and sweet stuff. Maybe I even drink a little too much. Therefore, I will change my diet, and quit sugar and liquor, except for a glass of red wine on the weekend.

As a Commander personality, I carry a lot of stress in my joints, too. For that, I am going to start asserting myself more at work, and maybe get a massage after the hot tub at the club once a week.

Diet: I will work with my first chakra by eating three balanced meals a day, with healthy proteins, lots of vegetables, vitamin B and C supplements, extra vitamin B_5, and liquid minerals. I am a goal setter. Now that I have decided this, I will do it. Fortunately, the Commander diet requirements are similar, but from that description, I will add more roughage by snacking on raw veggies and oil-free popcorn at work. I will also avoid all those "toxic foods," like bratwurst (except at a sports game), ham, and Chinese food with MSG. I will also drink more water.

Exercise: I will get a personal trainer to get me started. I will do weight lifting three times a week at the gym before work, making sure that I stretch, and get back to jogging twice a week, once on the weekend, when I have a lot more time.

Pitfalls and False Pleasures:
1. I overeat.
2. I love sweets and fatty foods.
3. As you say about Commanders, I get depressed more often than people think. I tell myself that I am nothing but a fat failure, and that my wife and children cannot possibly really love me.
4. Like many Commanders, I am judgmental. I think that I can run the department a lot better than my boss can. When he is being stupid, I get sarcastic.
5. I am ambitious, but do not know how to focus my energy to succeed. I am scared I will stop exercising because my joints hurt.

Success Tips: Here is how I will compensate for my weaknesses.
1. Because I overeat, like a lot of Commanders do, I will try that "eighty-five-bite" diet explained in the Thinker category. (Even though my Thinker scores are low, I think this is just because people said that I was "too dumb to succeed" because I was such a big kid.) I will eat eighty-five bites of food every day according to the "Diet Directives" program (see page 137).
2. I will eat one piece of dark chocolate every day for my sweet tooth, and eat salmon three times a week to fill up on "good" fats. The salmon will also help with the depression. Also, I will ask my wife to stop buying food low in nutritional content. If she and the children want it, they can go out for it.
3. I will get a mentor at my church to help me with my feelings of depression and to help me plan my career goals.
4. I will tune into my weak chakras of Feeler and Relater and do a "feelings check-in" with my wife every night. Maybe these chakras are low because I am really just scared of feelings.
5. I know that I *can* run the department better than my boss! I will start dressing for the position *ahead* of my boss and get my mentor to show me how to maneuver through the organization. I will not be so sarcastic to my boss. If I do want to say something unflattering to my boss, I will excuse myself and go to the bathroom.

6. I will get extra help by setting up an invisible board of directors, putting successful but deceased businesspeople on it. Every day, I will ask for business and body advice.
7. I will work with a chiropractor who specializes in Bio Energetic Synchronization Technique and uses an ARP machine (ask your chiropractor for more information), a process that repairs muscle injuries, to heal my joints and old football injuries.

Style: I can dress the part of my "future self," the self that I know that I can become, even before I have lost the seventy pounds around my middle. I will purchase two good suits immediately and take them in every fifteen pounds of weight drop. When I am at my goal, I will have a personal shopping assistant outfit me for success. Then I will "get groomed" at a good hair place, and keep my hair trim.

Supportive Assistants: Here is the help I will get:
1. Personal trainer
2. Massage therapist at the gym
3. Wife, for cooking and emotional support
4. Children, for help with keeping food low in nutritional content out of the house
5. Mentor through church
6. Invisible board of directors
7. Chiropractor
8. Hair dresser

Outcome: Anthony did it! Manifesters and Commanders are so goal-oriented that they often achieve their goals right on time, or even early. Anthony reached every objective. He lost weight, got closer to his wife, obtained a mentor, stuck to his exercise, bought his suits, and even got a promotion at work (in a different department, away from his boss). We then constructed a maintenance program, which included weekends away with his wife, work toward an MBA, a more intense workout, and increasing his per-meal bites from 85 to 115. Then we retested his chakra personality. His Feeler, Relater, and Thinker scores had increased! Childhood issues and cultural programming had previously overshadowed these inner assets. Now Anthony could bring them into the light and experience more light in his life.

CREATING YOUR PERFECT BODY PLAN

Complete the following statements to formulate your own body plan. You can use these statements whether you have a single or several strong chakras; simply summarize the main points of your strongest chakra personality descriptions to arrive at a synopsis.

Spiritual Requirements: This is the spiritual reason that I can work toward my perfect body:

Endocrine Effects: These are the special endocrine considerations I must keep in mind in order to unfold my perfect body:

Diet: Here are the most important components of my perfect body diet, including basic foods, special foods, number of meals daily, and supplements:

Exercise: My perfect body exercise plan includes these specific exercises and workout times:

Pitfalls and False Pleasures: These are my probable perfect body pitfalls:

Success Tips: These are my strategies for avoiding or minimizing my perfect body pitfalls and my tactics for assuring that I succeed at my perfect body plan:

Style: The following illustrates my optimum style, the look that reflects the self that I want to be in the future:

Supportive Assistants: These are people, energies, and energy exercises that will help me attract my perfect body:

Empowering Your Perfect Body:
The Four Forces

*Man is, in the full sense of the term, a 'miniature universe';
in him are all matters of which the universe consists; the
same forces, the same laws that govern the life of the universe,
operate in him; therefore in studying man we can study the
whole world, just as in studying the world we can study man.*

P.D. Ouspensky, *In Search of the Miraculous*

There are four forces in the universe. They have been described in many ways in many cultures, such as the four directions, the four elements, or the four aspects of our being. These four forces are also inherent in each of us, and they can be called upon to reinforce the perfecting of your body. Based upon my own assessment and best described in my book *Advanced Chakra Healing*, these forces and their chief characteristics are:

Force	Characteristic
Elemental	Physical
The Powers	Supernatural
Imagination	Magical
The Divine	Heavenly

Your strongest chakras excel at arresting and directing these four forces. You can draw on any of them to create your perfect body and attract additional universal energies that will make the job simple and joyful.

The Elemental Force

The physical world is reduced to millions of elements, all of which interact to create matter. Your body swirls with particles of dust and stars. It is empowered by fundamentals like fire and water and formulated by chemicals like nitrogen and oxygen. It is also fashioned from the realities of feeling and belief. Depending upon your chakra type, you access the specific elements that will encourage your spiritual mission and sustain your perfect body.

Individual chakras select elements appropriate to their functions based on frequency. A Naturalist will use the lowest-frequency energies, which most commonly relate to the color brown; natural substances like stone and earth; feelings and beliefs inherited from the ancestors; and spiritual philosophies that encompass the environment. Spiritualists will process higher-frequency elements, including those that emanate from the heavens. You will excel in pursuit of your perfect body by utilizing the elements that fit your personality type. When you use an element that matches your personality, the element transforms into a force that propels you at light speed toward your desired change.

The key to accessing elemental force is the power of intention. To make something happen with intention, you have to really mean it. You have to throw your entire being behind your goal, and keep going strong to the end. To accomplish this, you have to understand the potency of emotions.

Emotions are composed of beliefs paired with feelings. For instance, the belief "I deserve my perfect body" can serve as a testament to your dedication. It will keep you on target and positively motivated. Almost any feeling can be paired with a constructive belief like this one to assist you in effecting change. Anger will empower; fear will stimulate; sadness will heal; disgust will help you reject what is bad for you. Joy, however, is the strongest of all the feelings. When you couple joy with an affirming belief, you automatically bolster the effect of your belief tenfold, as long as you stay in the moment. You cannot imagine how happy you will be when you perfect your body. Feel how happy you are to have a body right now! Feel how thrilled you are to be strong enough to work your perfect body program today!

Every chakra draws upon different elements, can be imagined as a specific color, vibrates to a particular form of joy (which can also be seen as an awareness), and is most strongly upheld by certain positive beliefs. On the following page is a list of these characteristics. Note: The raw elements I work with include earth, stone, fire, water, wood, metal, air, light, ether, and star.

There are many ways to work elementally to support the emergence of your perfect body. For instance, you can imagine an element in your mind, selecting one associated with your strongest chakra. When under stress, such as when tempted by a pitfall, picture this element flooding your body, bolstering your will. Are you an eleventh-chakra person? Do you want to strengthen this chakra, or call upon the ability to command for change? Assert the power of the Commander inside by stating the belief listed on the above

Chakra	Raw Element	Color	Feeling or Awareness	Belief
First	Fire	Red	Passion	"I can do it"
Second	Water	Orange	Happiness	"I can create it"
Third	Wood	Yellow	Power of the mind	"My thoughts make it happen"
Fourth	Star	Green, Pink, or Gold	Love	"Love can do anything"
Fifth	Air	Blue	Truth	"Truth is power"
Sixth	Light	Purple	Possibilities	"What I see, I can become"
Seventh	Ether	White	Consciousness	"With conscious focus, I can create anything"
Eighth	All	Black or Silver	Power of knowledge	"My powers can create anything"
Ninth	Metal	Gold	Harmony	"The universe supports my goals"
Tenth	Earth	Brown	Needs are natural	"Nature supports my needs"
Eleventh	Stone	Rose	Forcefulness	"I can command anything and everything"

chart whenever possible. Are you a ninth-chakra maestro and feeling too guilty to eat nourishing foods, one of the pitfalls of being a ninth-chakra humanitarian? Ask the Divine to support you with the awareness of harmony, or infuse a metallic piece of jewelry with harmony energy to encourage a change of philosophy. Are you an eighth-chakra Shaman and having difficulty giving up coffee, one of your shamanic stimulants? Before drinking a coffee substitute, such as a grain-based beverage, imagine yourself swirling all ten elements into the drink, thus increasing its potency. Increase the effectiveness of this activity by imagining these elements as blending into the color silver, the color that reinforces your elemental strength. Would you like to access more elemental force? Wear or carry stones that reflect chakra elements (see page 137).

The Positive Side of Using the Elemental

By reducing your issues into their component building blocks you can restructure any part of your life. Are you overweight? Analyze what elements are "off." Decide which elements you need to accentuate, add the spice of feeling and the power of belief, and you can renovate each cell in your body! By focusing your feelings, awareness, and beliefs toward your end goal, you can obtain your perfect body one step at a time.

The Negative Side of Using the Elemental

It is difficult to determine all the factors contributing to each of your problems. Your insomnia, dislike of exercise, or hip problems might be attributable to hundreds of different factors. It is also difficult to stay focused on goals long enough to be completely effective.

THE POWER FORCE

Can you see the wind? We only perceive its existence when it blows off our hat, or perhaps the roof of our house. We know the wind exists because of the changes it produces. Like the wind, the power force is an invisible set of energies that motivate and shape the universe.

We are all able to summon power forces, usually through our strongest chakra centers. Would you like to encourage the healing properties of a supplemental herb or your soymilk, or flush toxins out of your system with a wish? Your chakras link to the powers of the universe, which stand by for your command.

Individual chakras specialize in different types of powers. Knowing the chakra-related powers can help you focus your mind when calling upon a power for a stated end. Ultimately, though, you do not have to name a power to use it, or specify which one you need. You only have to command the universe to send you the power required for a specific task. The Divine has established an orderly universe that automatically responds to your needs. This power is your spiritual right, and you exercise it through claiming your personal commanding powers.

It's important to know that you are vested with the intuitive knowledge of how to attract spiritual powers. By concentrating on your goal through the physical location of your strongest chakra, you marshal magical energies toward your desired end.

Here is an outline of each chakra, its physical location, and the verbal command that you can use to summon supernatural energies from beyond in order to support a specific or general body goal. A Feeler, for instance, might focus his consciousness in the abdomen (the location of the glands associated with the second chakra) and state the second chakra command, having already given implicit permission for the appropriate (and safe) power forces to enter his chakra center and carry out his desire. A Communicator will center in her thyroid, emphasize her need, and call forth the needed power. Try it and see for yourself!

First	
Chakra	Hips
Location	Adrenals
Power Command	"All physical energies will now focus to accomplish this goal"
Second	
Chakra	Abdomen
Location	Ovaries or testes
Power Command	"All creative forces now focus to accomplish this goal"
Third	
Chakra	Solar plexus
Location	Pancreas
Power Command	"All mental energies now organize so as to accomplish this goal"
Fourth	
Chakra	Heart
Location	Heart
Power Command	"I am so loved by the Divine; heaven and earth move to accomplish this goal"

Fifth	
Chakra	Throat
Location	Thyroid
Power Command	"I am speaking my desire, and all celestial energies converge to accomplish this goal"
Sixth	
Chakra	Forehead center
Location	Pituitary
Power Command	"I now attract all the spiritual energies needed to create my vision as reality"
Seventh	
Chakra	Top of the head
Location	Pineal
Power Command	"I have now attained the consciousness level necessary to allow the creation of this desire"
Eighth	
Chakra	One inch above the head
Location	Thymus
Power Command	"I now have the powers necessary to demand that the universe accomplish this task"
Ninth	
Chakra	One foot above the head
Location	Diaphragm
Power Command	"I am now in complete harmony with all, therefore allowing all of creation to deliver this desire"
Tenth	
Chakra	One foot below the feet
Location	Bones (such as sternum)
Power Command	"As a part of Nature, I now accept the gift of this goal from the Natural world"
Eleventh	
Chakra	Around the hands and feet
Location	Joints
Power Command	"As a creative force, I transmute all energies into positive forces and direct them to achieve this goal"

The Positive Side of Using the Power Force

Think of the Herculean results you can achieve by applying spiritual forces to your goals! Like a runner with rocket boosters on your shoes, you can accelerate your gains with a mere thought.

The Negative Side of Using the Power Force

Using power forces opens a host of ethical questions. If we can channel a supernatural energy through our first chakra and clear out toxic waste, can we then attack a hated neighbor with the same energy? It takes a lot of skill and a firm grasp on morality to apply the power properly.

THE IMAGINATION FORCE

In the beginning, there was the void. There were no books or airplanes, no televisions or motorcars. There were no walls upon which to display works of art; indeed, there were no artists to produce such works. And before the Creator could create? Before the words that summoned everything into being? There was an idea.

Everything concrete and solid began as an idea, the product of the imagination force. What situations resulted in you having your job? What preceded the purchase of your first car? The idea of what you wanted. Everything in reality began in someone's imagination. By better controlling your imagination process, you can more effectively transform your wishes into certainties.

How do you actualize the imagination force? Through your imagination, of course! Each chakra type will shine at certain ways of accessing the imagination. Use the method best for you and you can create miraculous and magical manifestations!

The next chart contains the methods of accessing the imagination related to each chakra, followed by examples of how each might be used.

Chakra	Methods of Accessing the Imagination
First	Action. Acknowledge your desire. Now act as if is you have already accomplished your goal.
Second	Feeling. Feel the feelings that you will experience once you have accomplished your goal.

Chakra	Methods of Accessing the Imagination
Third	Thinking. Form follows belief. Pretend that you have achieved your objective. What thoughts got you there? What belief accomplished this desire? Adopt this belief now.
Fourth	Relating. Imagine the types of relationships you will enjoy upon completing your task. How do you act? Live this way of loving immediately and your dreams will come true.
Fifth	Communicating. Manifesting through this chakra depends upon the words, tones, or intentions that we use to communicate with ourselves and the world. Imagine success. What messages created this success? Write down these messages and speak, sing, or think them from this moment forward.
Sixth	Visioning. Picture what you want, and what you will be like having received it. Picture the energies that caused you to achieve your goals every day and success will be yours.
Seventh	Consciousness. There are many levels of consciousness. Center your mind's eye in your pineal gland and sense the level of understanding or consciousness necessary to achieve your goals. Decide that from now on, this is the only level you will operate on. Your own consciousness will attract spiritual energies to materialize your goal.
Eighth	Knowledge. Do you know that you have the knowledge necessary to sway the universe to your bidding? To claim this authority, close your eyes and picture yourself performing the task or issuing the command that will bend the universe to your will. Ask your conscience or the Divine whether this goal or the method used is good for all affected or not. If not, ask for the proper goal or method.
Ninth	Harmonizing. Imagine that you have realized your dream. What did you need to believe, think, or feel to allow victory? Decide to accept the gift of success and it will be so.
Tenth	Mirroring. Everything that we want to receive or become is reflected in Nature. Abundance exists in the rain clouds; every drop of rain encourages the growth of crops. If you desire something, seek it in the natural world. Now ask the Great Spirit to invoke the spirit of that natural object, being, or life form to bring the same energies to you.
Eleventh	Authority. Do you know that you have the authority to transform energies at will? Know that the Divine has instilled this authority in you, and now use it! It does not matter whether you command with words, actions, pictures, or the briefest of glances. For the most ethical results, align first with divine will, as the Divine will then lend its powers to your own.

The Positive Side of Imagination

What if you could look in the mirror, imagine yourself slender and toned, and suddenly become so? Physics says that this is possible. Studies have shown that energy can move faster than the speed of light. In the space between two moments or thoughts, you can employ tachyon speed to rearrange matter. Imagination is a tool for manifesting changes, because it helps you perceive how you want things to be. Dream grandly to create something grand—including yourself.

The Negative Side of Imagination

Imagination has two steps. First, you imagine, or "make magic" in your mind. Second, you act magically, which implies taking action. Too many people dream big while sitting around getting bigger on chocolate bonbons. You have to move reality into being, not sit on it. Just believing does not make it so; you have to act.

THE DIVINE FORCE

Ultimately, all power comes from the Divine. In turn, the Divine grants us heavenly powers to accomplish our goals. These spiritual energies are vested in each chakra, but they are strongest in our major chakras. You do not need to be a full-fledged member of a particular church, synagogue, or mosque to gain the full support of the Divine. You do, however, need to apply the Divine force toward ends that further your authentic self, which includes the unfolding of your ideal body.

Each chakra is seeded with its own viewpoint about divine power. Focus on the spiritual truths of your strongest chakras when undertaking your perfect body plan and you will be amazed at the results.

The Positive Side of the Divine

Anything created through our divine abilities is good. There is no guilt, shame, or doubt when we manifest what God has already ordained. Claim your right to divine assistance and you will accelerate your progress toward success.

Chakra	Spiritual Truth
First	Physical and spiritual energies are the same; by meeting my physical needs, I become the spiritual being that the Divine intended me to be.
Second	Feelings reflect the places where we have accepted or not accepted unconditional love. I can follow my feelings and the Divine will use them to help me with my goals.
Third	My mind is one with God's mind. By holding only positive thoughts about myself and the world, I transform into my most positive self.
Fourth	There is nothing outside of love. By knowing that I am already unconditionally loved, I free myself from unhealthy patterns and behaviors.
Fifth	Reality is always composed of a greater truth (greater than is sometimes apparent). If I listen or speak only truth, I become the greater self that I am intended to be.
Sixth	The Divine sees me and sees only perfection. If I view myself through the eyes of the Divine, I will see everything that I need to achieve my greater goals.
Seventh	There is no such thing as a higher or lower consciousness, simply awareness of perfection. Because the Divine already sees me as perfect, I can become even more so by acting with love for myself.
Eighth	In some time or space, I have already done, thought, healed, or become everything needed to achieve my current goals. I can therefore draw upon my memories and powers to achieve my goals.
Ninth	Everything in the universe is already in harmony. By recognizing the harmonies in my current situation I create only more harmony, and therefore success.
Tenth	Nature is on the same order as heaven. Because I exist in Nature, I also exist in heaven, and can draw upon the miraculous powers of the heavenly to accomplish my goals.
Eleventh	Inner will and divine will are actually the same. I can set my will in accordance with the Divine, and divine force will empower everything I do.

The Negative Side of the Divine

There is nothing negative about the Divine, nor our use of divine forces. However, it is not always easy to believe in ourselves enough to co-create reality with the Divine. The Divine can breathe our wishes into being, but we must believe that we deserve to become what we really are.

YOUR PERFECT BODY

If I can give you one piece of advice, it would be this: Accept yourself. Your perfect body will emerge more quickly and with more ease if you accept the body that you now have.

Maybe you are dieting, exercising, and trying on a new style because you think that there is something wrong with your body as it is. Perhaps your nose is not suited for your face, or your body is not proportioned correctly. Maybe you hate your eyebrows or your lack of muscles. Maybe you even hate yourself. The truth is that you already live in your perfect body, simply because you are alive!

You already enjoy the capacity to laugh, linger over tea, eat mangoes at midnight, and even dance naked in the moonlight. Are you doing any of these things? Are you having fun in the body that you now occupy? It is okay to want a "better" body, to be healthier, fitter, sleeker, more tanned or toned. It's natural to want to crawl more nimbly on the floor with your children or the kittens next door. But don't wish away the body that you have in favor of one that doesn't yet exist on the physical plane.

The more able you are to love and accept the body that you *are*, the easier it will be to attract the loving, universal energies that can shape it into an even *more* perfect form. Perfect can simply become *perfect*. As you accept the self that you are, you allow yourself to become the even more amazing being that the Divine knows you to be.

Appendix

TACHYON SUCCESS: TIPS FOR ALL CHAKRA TYPES

For rapid health improvement and success, here are some strategies and resources that will accelerate your progress toward your perfect body.

For better nutrient absorption, try the Ziquin liquid supplement program: In general, it is always best to select liquid minerals and vitamins. Unlike solid supplements, liquid supplements don't have to be processed by the stomach first. Because they are absorbed in your mouth, they reach the bloodstream faster.

The best all-around liquid supplement program I have discovered is Ziquin, a five-part, daily process that is customized to your individual nutritional needs. Ziquin supplements are specifically formulated for absorption and stability. For more information and ordering, see www.ziquin.com.

To improve overall homeostasis and well-being, consider BioSET bioenergetic testing and enzyme therapy. BioSET is a computerized approach to the Oriental meridian system that aims to improve strength and vitality. Pain-free, it is an excellent, noninvasive way to test for the presence of allergies, diseases, and emotional issues as underlying causes of health issues. See www.bioset.net.

To improve psychological and psychosomatic stability, consider Eye Movement Desensitization and Reprocessing (EMDR). I recommend professional psychotherapy that features EMDR because it allows you to pinpoint and clear the causes of psychological and behavioral problems, including allergies, food issues, depression, and anxiety. Practitioners skilled in this practice can help you change your neurological patterns in a relatively short amount of time. For more information, please refer to www.emdr.com.

For injuries, consider Matrix Repatterning. This relatively new practice is a hands-on healing modality that seeks to restructure cellular walls damaged by accidents, falls, surgery, and other physical trauma. For more information and lists of practitioners, see www.rothinstitute.com.

For help controlling dietary intake, check out the Diet Directives program. Diet Directives helps you limit the amount of food you eat by encouraging you to eat eighty-five bites a day—no more, no less. For more information, see www.dietdirectives.com.

For energy support, consider crystal therapy. Rocks, crystals, and metals transmit energy, release toxic elements, and attract supportive energies. Use the crystals of the color of your main chakras and you will boost the effectiveness of that chakra to attract your perfect body. Refer to a crystal therapy book for more information, such as *The Crystal Bible* by Judy Hall (Godsfield Press).

For a healthy sugar substitute, use Stevia powder. Stevia is an extraordinarily sweet herb that is 200 to 300 times sweeter than sugar. It has been used as a sweetener for thousands of years by native people in South America, where it grows wild. Almost calorie-free, it is beneficial for weight reduction because, unlike sugar, it doesn't trigger a rise in blood sugar. It is a good substitute for table sugar and for Nutrasweet, which can trigger allergic reactions in many people. Stevia is available in whole leaf, powder, and liquid forms, including one for cooking, and is now available at most grocery and health food stores.

Notes

1. Hunbatz Men, *Secrets of Mayan Science/Religion* (Santa Fe: Bear & Company, 1990), p. 27.
2. Roger Williams Ph.D., *Biochemical Individuality: The Basis for the Genetotropic Concept* (New Canaan, CT: Keats Publishing, 1999).
3. Brenda Kearns, "Think Yourself Healthy," *Woman's World*, October 5, 2004, p. 12.